PICKARD'S MANUAL OF
OPERATIVE DENTISTRY

PICKARD'S MANUAL OF
Operative Dentistry

Seventh Edition

•

E. A. M. KIDD

Professor of Cariology,
United Medical and Dental School,
Guy's Hospital, London

AND

B. G. N. SMITH

Professor of Conservative Dentistry,
United Medical and Dental School,
Guy's Hospital, London

IN COLLABORATION WITH

H. M. PICKARD

Emeritus Professor in Conservative Dentistry,
University of London,
Formerly of the Royal Dental Hospital of London,
School of Dental Surgery

Oxford   New York   Tokyo
OXFORD UNIVERSITY PRESS
1996

Oxford University Press, Walton Street, Oxford OX2 6DP
Oxford New York
Athens Auckland Bangkok Bombay
Calcutta Cape Town Dar es Salaam Delhi
Florence Hong Kong Istanbul Karachi
Kuala Lumpur Madras Madrid Melbourne
Mexico City Nairobi Paris Singapore
Taipei Tokyo Toronto
and associated companies in
Berlin Ibadan

Oxford is a trade mark of Oxford University Press

Published in the United States
by Oxford University Press Inc., New York

A catalogue record for this book is available from the British Library

Library of Congress Cataloging in Publication Data
Kidd, Edwina A. M.
*Pickard's manual of operative dentistry.—7th ed./E. A. M. Kidd
and B. G. N. Smith; in collaboration with H. M. Pickard.*
p. cm. —(Oxford medical publications)
Includes bibliographical references and index.
*1. Dentistry, Operatives. I. Pickard, H. M. (Hula Masters)
II. Smith, Bernard G. N. III. Title. IV. Title: Manual of
operative dentistry. V. Series.*
[DNLM: 1. Dentistry, Operative. WU 300 P594m 1996]
RK501.P64 1996 617.6'7—dc20 95–10505
DNLM/DLC for Library of Congress
ISBN 0 19 262610 8 (Hbk)
ISBN 0 19 262609 4 (Pbk)

Typeset by Cotswold Typesetting Ltd, Gloucester
Printed and bound in Hong Kong

FOREWORD TO THE SIXTH EDITION

THE fact that *A manual of operative dentistry* is now in its sixth edition is testimony to the contribution that Professor Pickard has made to undergraduate teaching. I have known him for nearly 40 years and during his teaching career he was always ready to try out new materials and techniques and advance the frontiers of dental science. Not for him the ultra-conservative approach to new ideas that can often kill the younger undergraduate teacher's enthusiasm for dentistry. The originality of his two new co-authors, Bernard Smith and Edwina Kidd, assures the continuity of his work. The student is certain to enjoy this new edition since it moves on to new ground in which prevention, minimal mechanical intervention, and adhesive bonding of materials to teeth challenge the old concepts of cavity preparation and just filling a tooth with an amalgam plug. This book allows the student reader to start his clinical career in restorative dentistry with a sound knowledge of this new thinking. The book is well planned and the reader is taken through a logical sequence of clinical diagnosis and treatment from 'Why restore teeth?' to the more complex forms of cast metal and porcelain intracoronal restorations. The student is given a vision of what is required in maintaining a dentition from the relatively simple procedures described in this book to the future postgraduate education required to become a master in both fixed and removable prosthodontics. In particular, the opening chapters weave a thread of common sense which reflects, in particular, Edwina Kidd's outstanding work on the treatment of the early carious lesion. As each chapter unfolds the student is made more and more aware that the carious lesion is a process of destruction and repair and needs treating accordingly. The authors have wisely stayed away from the dogma surrounding early caries treatment and avoided falling between the stools of 'over-prescription' or 'supervised neglect'. The student reader is given a sensible start to his career which I think reflects the situation in general practice. The later chapters on the more complex forms of treatment are refreshing for their rational approach to the somewhat over-enthusiastic adoption of new technologies such as the porcelain veneer or bonded porcelain inlay. The hand of Bernard Smith can be seen here in which the student is encouraged to adopt this new technology but to use it wisely in the right clinical situation and be aware of the difficulties that are encountered as skills are developed. Long-lasting restorative dentistry builds practices and although patients only begin to appreciate high-quality dentistry with the passage of time, the future rewards for the undergraduate are not only monetary but also include that well-worn phrase 'job satisfaction'. As each decade goes by in general practice it is easy to slip into a routine in the surgery. Postgraduate education and an ability to retain enthusiasm for new ideas will keep the undergraduate intellectually refreshed and a better practitioner of his art and science.

This book, although primarily aimed at the undergraduate, is also well suited to the practising dentist. The authors are to be congratulated on writing a book that unifies much of our current thinking in restorative dentistry and sets a pattern for undergraduate education in the next decade.

JOHN W. MCLEAN, OBE
FDS, MDS, DSC (Lond.), D.ODONT. (Lund.)
Clinical Consultant, Laboratory of the Government Chemist,
38 Devonshire Street, London W1N 1LD
March 1989

PREFACE TO THE SEVENTH EDITION

At Professor Pickard's request the sixth edition of this book was a major revision of the text. By comparison, the changes to the seventh edition are less substantial but nevertheless include a significant amount of new text and new illustrations to bring the book up to date. This has necessitated some changes to virtually every page, and some sections have been completely revised. The speed with which the subject advances is a testament to the ingenuity and enthusiasm of the profession.

The main changes in this edition include further consideration of caries risk, the mechanisms of pulpal pathology and the diagnosis of erosive toothwear. There is more on the clinically relevant materials science of amalgam, composite, glass ionomer cements, including the newer resin-modified glass ionomer materials, and dentine-bonding agents. The 'amalgam controversy' is discussed.

In the chapters on treatment technique more emphasis has been placed on layered glass ionomer—composite restorations and descriptions of the use of amalgam for the management of smooth surface lesions have been deleted, not because of concern about amalgam but because we now consider that the new materials are superior in these situations.

Recommendations on the need for replacement of restorations have been made more definitive, based on recent research findings. However, as in the previous editions every effort has been made to point out areas of ignorance in the hope that this text will serve as a basis for discussion rather than a solid tablet of stone.

Those photographs not taken by the authors are the work of Usha Desai whose skill is clearly seen in the following pages. We are very grateful to her.

We are also considerably indebted to several colleagues who have lent us illustrations. They are acknowledged in the captions to the relevant figures together with the source of the original publication where applicable.

September 1995

E.A.M.K.
B.G.N.S.
H.M.P.

PREFACE TO THE SIXTH EDITION

THE first five editions of this book have served a succession of undergraduate dental students and dental practitioners for over a quarter of a century. In that time great advances have been made in the understanding of dental disease and its management, and in restorative materials and the techniques by which they are used.

Prevention of dentistry's most prevalent diseases, though far from complete, has reached a stage of reality which only the most optimistic dared predict a few decades ago. Silver amalgam after one and a half centuries of use—and, it must be admitted, misuse—is still, in spite of its obvious shortcomings, the most widely used posterior restorative material. But it is increasingly being overtaken by other materials having new and continually developing properties, opening up avenues of technical ingenuity and advance.

Many of these changes have been incorporated in previous editions but there comes a time when such periodical updating is no longer adequate because the philosophical basis of modern clinical practice has moved on; so too has that of clinical teaching. A useful textbook employing the best media of graphic communication must reflect these changes, giving clear and unambiguous guidance to the student and food for thought to the experienced practitioner. This edition has undergone thorough reorganization of the text to take advantage of the changing pattern of teaching from a technique-orientated approach to one of disease control and clinical problem solving.

This change in rationale is represented by dividing the book into three parts. The first and last are primarily concerned with decision making, always important, but even more so now when the choice is greater and the immediate and remote consequences of restoring or not restoring teeth are better understood. The second part deals with treatment techniques which are just as important as they ever were but which must be seen within the overall context of patient management.

To emphasize this, Chapters 6–9 each deal with a clinical problem and consider the range of techniques which may be used to solve it. For instance Chapter 6 covers occlusal caries and the management techniques range from fissure sealing to the large occlusal restorations in amalgam or composite.

In a few instances we have included, with caution, techniques of which the logic is based upon the special properties of newer materials used in a specific manner. Their purpose is usually to favour conservation of sound tissue. The final judgement on the value of these procedures has yet to be made for it depends upon the essential test of prolonged exposure to clinical conditions. On present evidence anticipation of good results seems justified. In these conditions a well-balanced choice may be needed if we are to heed Alexander Pope's counsel:

> Be not the first by whom the new are tried,
> Nor yet the last to lay the old aside.

At a time when technology is developing so rapidly we do well to keep our minds open to new and better applications wherever they may be found.

Another innovation is the replacement of most of the line drawings by clinical colour photographs and step-by-step illustration of the most important procedures. Practical dentistry is complicated and difficult, and line drawings sometimes oversimplify the problems so that the student trying to follow the technique does not understand why he or she is not succeeding. The very high quality of modern colour photography and reproduction now allow us to show real problems in real teeth. This realism more than compensates the advantages a drawing may have. We hope our readers will feel that this is a valuable step toward showing dentistry as it is.

When this book was first written the choice of simple undergraduate texts was limited and so it was necessary to include relatively brief reference to extracoronal restorations and endodontics. These topics are now well covered by other books and they have been omitted from this edition rather than fail to do them justice.

London   E.A.M.K.
March 1989   B.G.N.S.
                                                                                          H.M.P.

CONTENTS

PART II
TREATMENT TECHNIQUES

PART I

DISEASES, DISORDERS, DIAGNOSES, DECISIONS, AND DESIGN

1   Why restore teeth?

THE four conditions which result in defective tooth structure, sometimes requiring repair, are dental caries, tooth wear, trauma, and developmental defects. This chapter discusses the aetiology, prevention, diagnosis, and management of these conditions.

A clear understanding of such aspects of these conditions as the time-scale involved, the histological changes, the permanence or otherwise of the change, and the symptoms or other effects they cause are essential if the dentist is to plan and execute treatment logically, effectively, and in the patient's best interests. Indeed, the dentist will need the information to decide whether treatment is necessary at all.

DENTAL CARIES

Dental caries is a disease of the calcified tissues of the teeth caused by the action of micro-organisms on fermentable carbohydrates. It is characterized by demineralization of the mineral portion of enamel and dentine followed by disintegration of their organic material. As the disease approaches the pulp, it produces changes in the form of reactionary dentine and pulpitis (possibly giving pain), and may result in bacterial invasion and death of the pulp. The infected necrotic pulp then produces further changes in the periapical tissues.

On the other hand, the disease can be arrested in its early stages since it is possible for remineralization to occur. In addition, progress of the disease to a clinical cavity is not inevitable, and can be completely prevented by relatively simple measures.

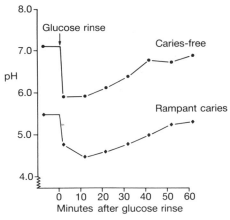

Fig. 1.1 Changes in pH in plaque following a glucose rinse ('Stephan curve').

Aetiology of dental caries

Four factors are necessary to produce dental caries:

- dental plaque

- a suitable carbohydrate (mainly sugar)

- a susceptible tooth surface

- time.

These factors work together in the following way. Some *plaque bacteria* are capable of fermenting a suitable *dietary carbohydrate substrate* (such as the sugars sucrose and glucose) to produce acid, causing the plaque pH to fall within 1–3 minutes. Unfortunately the plaque remains acid for some time, taking 30–60 minutes to return to its normal pH in the region of 7. This change in plaque pH can be represented graphically over a period of time following a glucose rinse (Fig. 1.1). It is such repeated falls in pH which *in time* may result in demineralization of *a susceptible tooth surface*, thus initiating the carious process. The interplay of these factors can be represented diagrammatically (Fig. 1.2). Only when all four factors are present will caries occur.

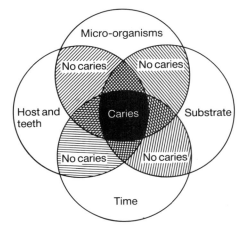

Fig. 1.2 The four circles represent the interplay of the aetiological factors in dental caries. All four factors must be acting simultaneously for caries to occur.

Susceptible sites

Since caries is caused by bacterial plaque, the following sites on the tooth surface which favour plaque retention and stagnation are particularly prone to decay.

- Enamel pits and fissures on occlusal surfaces of molar and premolar teeth (Fig. 1.3); buccal pits of molars and palatal pits of maxillary incisors.

- Approximal enamel smooth surfaces just cervical to the contact area (Fig. 1.4).

- The enamel at the cervical margin of the tooth at the gingival margin (Fig. 1.5). In patients with gingival recession, the area of plaque stagnation is on the exposed root surface (Fig. 1.6).

- The margins of restorations, particularly those where there is a gap between the restoration and the tooth or those where the restoration overhangs the margin of the cavity (Fig. 1.7).

Fig. 1.3

Fig. 1.4

Fig. 1.5

Fig. 1.3   Occlusal caries in a lower first molar tooth.

Fig. 1.4   A carious lesion is present on the distal aspect of the first premolar tooth. The lesion is shining through the marginal ridge which shows a pinkish grey discoloration.

Fig. 1.5   White spot enamel lesions at the cervical margins of both molar teeth.

Fig. 1.6   Caries on the exposed buccal root surface of the first premolar tooth.

Fig. 1.7   Caries at the margin of the occlusal restoration in the first molar tooth.

Fig. 1.6

Fig. 1.7

The first three sites are listed in the order of frequency in which caries develops. Thus, pit and fissure caries is more common than approximal caries and, at least in younger age groups before gingival recession becomes common, buccal and lingual caries at the cervical margin is the least common. However, in older patients root surfaces exposed by gingival recession may be the predominant site for caries to occur. The frequency of caries at the fourth site—secondary caries around restorations (see p. 184)—should be, in a perfect world, the least common. However, it is not, for reasons which will be discussed in Chapter 11.

Site susceptibility will be affected by local factors such as irregular or overlapping teeth, and areas where access is difficult for cleaning such as around the distal-buccal surface of upper second and third molar teeth.

Severity or rapidity of attack

Under normal conditions the tooth is continually bathed in saliva which is capable of remineralizing the early carious lesion because it is supersaturated with calcium and phosphate ions. This means that the carious process consists of alternating periods of destruction and repair, and for this reason caries does not destroy the tooth in days or weeks but rather in months or years. Since the disease can be arrested in its early stages, there is a good deal of scope for preventive measures.

Dental caries may be classified according to the severity or rapidity of the attack, and different teeth and surfaces are involved depending on the severity. Thus in a mild case only the most vulnerable teeth and surfaces are attacked, such as occlusal pits and fissures. A moderate attack may involve occlusal and approximal surfaces of posterior teeth and in a severe attack anterior teeth, which otherwise remain caries-free, also become carious. This introduces the concept of *individual variation of teeth*. In addition, *patients* vary in their susceptibility to the disease; in managing dental caries it is essential to fit the treatment to the needs of the individual patient.

Rampant caries

Rampant caries is the term used to describe a sudden rapid destruction of many teeth, frequently involving surfaces of teeth that are ordinarily relatively caries-free. Rampant caries is most commonly observed in the primary dentition of infants who continually suck a bottle or comforter containing, or dipped into, a sugar solution (Fig. 1.8). Rampant caries may also be seen in the permanent dentition of teenagers and is usually due to frequent cariogenic snacks and sweet drinks between meals (Fig. 1.9). It is also seen in mouths where there is a sudden marked reduction in salivary flow (xerostomia). Radiation in the region of the salivary glands, used in the treatment of a malignant growth, is the most common cause of severe xerostomia. In addition, a large number of therapeutic drugs, such as antidepressants, tranquillizers, antihypertensives, and diuretics, retard salivary flow.

Fig. 1.8 Rampant caries of the deciduous teeth. This child continuously sucked a bottle of sweet drink.

The management of rampant caries is more difficult than the management of caries which has progressed at a slower pace because of the extent of the caries and the rate at which it progresses. However, the treatment is the same in principle. The disease is managed by preventing further disease and stabilizing existing lesions before restoring teeth permanently. If caries is not managed preventively, the restorative treatment will be doomed to a cycle of disease, repair, new disease and further repair, and, before too long, extraction.

Fig. 1.9 Rampant caries in a 19-year-old man.

Arrested caries

Arrested caries is in distinct contrast to rampant caries, and the term describes carious lesions which do not progress. It is seen when the oral environment has changed from conditions predisposing to caries to conditions that tend to slow the lesion down. Figure 1.10 shows an arrested lesion on the mesial aspect of a lower second molar. The lesion probably stopped after extraction of the first molar. The environment changed, becoming easier to clean and more accessible to saliva. Operative treatment is clearly not necessary.

The carious process in enamel

The earliest clinically visible evidence of enamel caries is the white spot lesion, for example at the cervical margin of the tooth (Fig. 1.5). This may also be seen on extracted teeth as a small opaque white area just cervical to where the approximal contact area was. The colour of the lesion distinguishes it from the adjacent sound enamel, but at this stage there is no cavity and the enamel overlying the white spot is hard and often shiny. Sometimes the lesion may appear brown due to exogenous stains absorbed by this porous region. Both white and brown spot lesions may have been present in the mouth for some years, as it is not inevitable for a carious lesion to progress.

Fig. 1.10 Arrested caries on the mesial aspect of the second molar tooth. This lesion probably stopped progressing after extraction of the first molar tooth.

Fig. 1.11 Longitudinal ground section through a carious lesion on a smooth surface examined in water with polarized light. The lesion is cone-shaped. Note the relatively intact surface zone (SZ).

Fig. 1.12 A longitudinal ground section through an occlusal fissure showing a small carious lesion in enamel. The section is in water and viewed in polarized light. The lesion forms on the fissure walls, giving the appearance of two smooth surface lesions.

If this smooth surface early lesion is examined histologically in a ground section with transmitted light, it is usually seen to be cone-shaped, with the apex of the cone pointing towards the enamel-dentine junction (Fig. 1.11). One of the most important features of the histological picture is that the early enamel lesion is a subsurface demineralization beneath a relatively intact surface zone.

Why caries should develop in this way has been a puzzle for many years. If acid is applied directly to enamel, the surface tissue is etched away in quite a different way from the subsurface demineralization characteristic of caries. It appears that dental plaque is principally responsible for this appearance, trapping calcium and phosphate ions released by subsurface dissolution and allowing them to reprecipitate into the enamel surface. Thus, the histological appearance of the relatively intact surface zone emphasizes that caries is not simply a process of demineralization but an alternating process of destruction and repair. However, if the early enamel lesion progresses, the intact surface breaks down, forming a hole (cavitation). This is no longer reversible by remineralization since actual cavities will not fill up from the base.

Plaque formation continues within the cavity and may not be accessible to cleaning aids such as a toothbrush or dental floss. For this reason a cavitated lesion is more likely to progress, although it can still become arrested and, where the basic structure remains, partially remineralize.

Fissures and pits are obvious stagnation areas where plaque can form and mature, anatomically protected from the toothbrush filament by the dimensions of the fissure.

The histological features of fissure caries are similar to those already described for smooth surfaces. The lesion forms around the fissure walls and gives the appearance in section of two small smooth surface lesions (Fig. 1.12). Eventually the lesions increase in size, broadening and coalescing at the base of the fissure.

The carious process in dentine

If the carious process reaches the enamel-dentine junction, caries spreads laterally along it to involve the dentine on a wider front. This results in sound enamel being undermined, and the resulting lesion is larger than would be expected from examination of the enamel alone, particularly in fissure lesions (Fig. 1.13).

Undermined enamel is brittle and will in due course fracture if subjected to occlusal forces, producing a large cavity. Undermined enamel is of particular relevance in cavity preparation because superficially sound but undermined enamel must often be removed to gain access to carious dentine beneath it. In addition, it is

Fig. 1.13 (a) An upper molar with a stained fissure. (b) A hemisection of this tooth showing a larger dentine lesion than would be expected from examination of the enamel alone.

(a)

(b)

probably unwise to leave undermined enamel occlusally unless it is supported by a restorative material that adheres to it, because the forces of occlusion may fracture it. For these reasons the extent of lateral spread of caries along the enamel-dentine junction is one of the main determinants of the size of a prepared cavity.

Pulp–dentine defence reactions

Dentine is a vital tissue containing the cytoplasmic extensions of the odontoblasts and must be considered together with the pulp since the two tissues are so intimately connected. The pulp-dentine complex, like any other vital tissue in the body, is capable of defending itself. The state of the tissue at any time will depend on the balance between the attacking forces and the defence reactions. The important defence reactions are tubular sclerosis within the dentine, reactionary dentine at the interface between dentine and pulp, and inflammation of the pulp.

Tubular sclerosis occurs through precipitation of minerals in the tubular space and is protective in that it reduces the permeability of the dentine, inhibiting the penetration of acids and bacterial toxins. Reactionary dentine is formed by the odontoblasts beneath the carious stimulus. A slowly progressing small lesion may give time for a considerable reparative dentine response, whereas with more acute larger lesions the response may be disorganized or even non-existent. This retreat of the pulp from injury has important implications in the operative management of caries (see p. 50).

Inflammation is the fundamental response of all vascular connective tissues to injury. Inflammation of the pulp (pulpitis) may, as in any other tissue, be acute or chronic. In a slowly progressing carious lesion, toxins reaching the pulp may provoke chronic inflammation. However, once the organisms actually reach the pulp (a carious exposure), acute inflammation may supervene.

Inflammatory reactions have vascular and cellular components. In chronic inflammation the cellular components predominate and there may be increased collagen production, leading to fibrosis but without immediately endangering the vitality of the tooth. However, in acute inflammation the vascular changes predominate.

Infection is the most common cause of pulpal inflammation and caries is the most common microbial source. Caries of peripheral dentine will result in pulpal inflammation and chronic inflammatory cells (macrophages, lymphocytes, and plasma cells) will infiltrate the pulp near the odontoblast layer. Indeed, this infiltration may even be seen in initial enamel caries. This chronic inflammatory reaction is mainly due to the movement of bacterial toxins through the dentinal tubules. With increasing carious involvement of enamel and dentine, the area of chronic inflammation increases in size but it is believed to remain localized until pulp exposure. After exposure, bacteria may enter the pulp. Polymorphonuclear leucocytes may now predominate, and acute inflammation can supervene and spread throughout the pulp, resulting in pulpal necrosis.

One objective of the preparation of a carious cavity for a filling is to remove bacterial infection before carious exposure occurs. Once the bacterial irritant is removed, the local inflammation it has caused has an inherent potential to heal provided that the cavity is restored with a non-irritating material that seals the margin of the filling. This cavity seal prevents further bacterial ingress and assault on the pulp–dentine complex.

However, if the irritants are not completely removed, or if the operative procedure is performed in a manner that is harmful to the pulp or the restorative material is irritating or defective, a local necrosis in the pulp can result. The area of necrosis may harbour bacteria and the inflammation may move apically until the entire pulp is necrotic. This is followed either by spread of toxins into the periapical tissues at the root apex, producing the chronic inflammatory response of chronic apical periodontitis, or, if organisms pass into the periapical tissues, an acute apical abscess develops (see pp. 43, 44).

Degenerative or destructive changes in dentine

These include demineralization of dentine, destruction of the organic matrix, and damage and death of odontoblasts. Since carious enamel is porous, acids, enzymes, and other chemical stimuli from the tooth surface will reach the outer dentine, evoking a response in the pulp-dentine complex. Thus, both reparative and degenerative changes begin before cavitation of the enamel occurs and while the micro-organisms are still confined to the tooth surface. With cavitation of enamel, bacteria have direct access to dentine and the tissue becomes infected.

Demineralization of dentine precedes bacterial penetration, and this is of great importance in operative dentistry since a major objective is to remove the infected and necrotic dentine, although uninfected but demineralized dentine may be left in some circumstances.

Of course, this is easier said than done because it is difficult to differentiate between the two layers. Thus, where the pulp is not at risk or the strength of the tooth is not jeopardized, all the carious dentine is removed. However, if the carious dentine is close to the pulp, it is often left if it is reasonably hard, even though it may contain a few organisms. It is treated with a lining material with a high pH, in an attempt to counteract the effect of the organisms, to seal them from their supply of nutrients, and to allow reparative dentine formation. This is discussed further in Chapters 3 and 7.

It is important to realize that the rate of progress of caries in dentine is highly variable and under suitable environmental conditions the progress of the disease can be arrested. Clinically, actively progressing lesions are soft, and, because of the speed at which some lesions develop, the defence reactions may not have time to be effective. In contrast, arrested or slowly progressing lesions have a hard, leathery, or dry consistency. The defence reactions are well marked and the carious lesion accumulates minerals from the oral fluids.

Root caries

Dentine caries beneath enamel has been considered in the preceding section. However, root surfaces become exposed in many mouths and these surfaces are susceptible to root caries and also appear more vulnerable than enamel to mechanical wear and chemical damage (see p. 20).

Exposed root surfaces occur following gingival recession, which is usually associated with periodontal disease, and so it is hardly surprising that root caries is more commonly seen in older people. Not all patients with exposed root surfaces will automatically contract root caries since a cariogenic plaque and diet are also required.

Histologically, in the early lesion demineralization appears to take place beneath a well-mineralized surface layer. Deep to the lesion there are often areas of tubular sclerosis and reactionary dentine. Bacteria seem to penetrate the tissues at an earlier stage in root caries than in coronal caries, although lesions are often rather superficial.

Clinically, both active (soft) and arrested lesions or slowly progressing lesions (hard) may be seen. Active lesions are commonly seen adjacent to the gingival margin.

Secondary or recurrent caries

Placing a restoration does not confer immunity on the tooth, and secondary or recurrent caries may occur in the tooth tissue adjacent to the filling material.

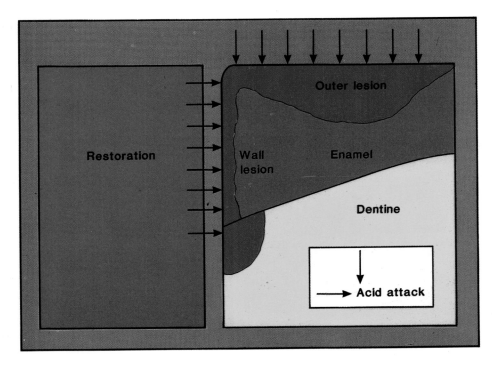

Fig. 1.14 A diagrammatic representation of secondary caries. The lesion may occur in two parts: an 'outer lesion' formed on the surface of the tooth as a result of primary attack, and a 'cavity wall lesion' formed as a result of leakage between the restoration and the cavity wall.

When a coronal filling is placed, the adjacent enamel can be considered in two planes—the surface enamel and the enamel of the cavity wall. For this reason a secondary carious lesion has been described as occurring in two parts (Fig. 1.14)— an *outer lesion* formed on the surface of the tooth as a result of primary attack, and a cavity *wall lesion* which will only be seen if bacteria and fluids, or at least hydrogen ions originating from plaque on the surface, leak into the microspace between the restoration and the cavity wall.

An enormous amount of research effort has been devoted to finding filling materials which will hermetically seal the cavity and thus prevent development of the wall lesion. These attempts have not been entirely successful but results of investigations with some more recently developed materials, such as the glass ionomer cements, are encouraging. However, many restorations exhibit marginal leakage and in a caries-prone mouth any restoration may fail through secondary caries.

This emphasizes the point that the best way of managing caries is by prevention and not by filling holes in teeth. Even the very best operative dentistry is a poor substitute for unblemished enamel and dentine, and operative dentistry must be seen as making good a failure to prevent disease from occurring or progressing in the first place.

DIAGNOSIS OF DENTAL CARIES

Early diagnosis of the carious lesion has become even more important since the realization that caries is not simply a process of demineralization but an alternating process of destruction and repair. Saliva is an excellent remineralizing fluid and the balance can be tipped in favour of repair by modifying diet, careful use of fluoride, and removing plaque (see p. 17).

The earlier caries can be diagnosed the better since small lesions will remineralize more readily than large ones, and a cavity is in some ways a point of no return since holes in the dental tissues are not expected to calcify up from the base. However, a cavitated lesion will not necessarily progress, and so an important question for the practitioner to answer is: What will become arrested and what must be repaired by restoration?

The diagnostic procedure

The diagnosis of caries requires good lighting and dry clean teeth. If heavy deposits of calculus or plaque are present, the mouth should be cleaned before attempting accurate diagnosis. Each quadrant of the mouth should be isolated in turn with cotton-wool rolls and dried with air or cotton-wool pledgets.

Sharp eyes are used to look for the earliest signs of disease, and vision can be enhanced by the use of magnification. Magnifying loupes can be worn on a head band or attached to spectacles. Alternatively, special glasses with telescopes attached can be used, and, although expensive, have the advantage that they can be made to a specific focal length to suit the particular operator. Operative dentistry can only be made easier by the use of magnification (see p. 86). Traditionally a sharp probe was used to detect caries in enamel either by the rough feel of early cavitation on a smooth surface, or by the probe tips wedging between the softened sides of a fissure. This was known as a 'sticky fissure'. However, a sharp probe can damage an incipient carious lesion, actually causing cavitation in a lesion which might otherwise have arrested (Fig. 1.15). Further, by carrying micro-organisms into the lesion a probe may facilitate the spread of the carious process. Therefore a probe should not be used in the diagnosis of enamel caries.

Good bite-wing radiographs are essential for some sites. The central X-ray beam is directed at right angles to the long axis of the teeth, and tangentially through the contact areas at a film positioned intra-orally on the lingual side of the posterior teeth. The film should be held in a film-holder which is attached to a beam-aiming device. This allows accurate positioning of the tube (Fig 1.16). Film-holders and beam-aiming devices take the guesswork out of positioning the X-ray beam at right angles to the film. They also make it possible to take the same view on a subsequent occasion, allowing the films to be compared (see p. 17).

Diagnosis of caries in pits and fissures

Caries in pits and fissures is difficult to diagnose at an early stage since the lesion forms in the depth of the fissure and cannot readily be seen. A probe may be used gently to remove any plaque from the fissure but should not be pressed into the fissure. Clinical diagnosis is primarily by vision, looking for surface discoloration, cavitation, and the grey appearance of enamel undermined by caries (Fig. 1.3).

A frank cavity, or hole in the occlusal enamel, is a relatively late presentation of the carious process. Such lesions always require operative repair. However, it is important to realize that large lesions may be present in dentine with no cavity in the outer enamel. Indeed, sometimes the surface of the tooth looks completely healthy, but demineralization may be present in the dentine. These lesions are called 'hidden' or 'occult' caries. It has been suggested that occlusal caries has become more difficult to diagnose since the advent of fluoride toothpaste because the fluoride encourages enamel remineralization, concealing lesion progression in the dentine beneath. Scientific evidence that this is really a new phenomenon is lacking, but contemporary clinicians agree that occlusal caries often cannot be diagnosed by vision alone. For this reason, bite-wing radiographs are of great importance in the detection of occlusal caries *in dentine*, although enamel caries cannot be seen. By the time that a lesion can be seen radiographically it is well into dentine (Fig. 1.17) and a restoration is required.

Fig. 1.15 A smooth surface lesion before and after probing. Note the damage that can be caused by a sharp probe.

Fig. 1.16 A film-holder and beam-aiming device in use to take a bite-wing radiograph.

Fig. 1.17 A bite-wing radiograph showing occlusal caries in the lower second molar tooth (arrow). Clinically there was no detectable cavity in this tooth, although the fissure was stained and the enamel discoloured.

Therefore early diagnosis of caries in pits and fissures is difficult, and the anatomy of the area favours lesion spread rather than lesion arrest. These facts are of considerable relevance in the management of the disease and are discussed further in Chapter 6.

Diagnosis of caries on approximal surfaces

As with the fissure, it is difficult to see the 'early' carious enamel lesion on an approximal surface. This is because the lesion forms just cervical to the contact area and vision is obscured by the adjacent tooth. If the lesion is discovered clinically, it is usually at a relatively late stage when it has already progressed well into dentine and is seen as a pinkish grey area shining up through the marginal ridge (Fig. 1.4). It must be emphasized again that teeth should be isolated, clean, and dry to pick up this appearance.

Bite-wing radiographs are of paramount importance in diagnosing approximal caries *in both enamel and dentine* (Fig. 1.18). However, it should be remembered that the technique is relatively insensitive, and once a lesion is visible in enamel on a bite-wing radiograph it is usually in dentine when examined histologically.

The approximal enamel lesion appears as a dark triangular area in the enamel on a bite-wing radiograph. The lesion may be seen just in the outer enamel, throughout the depth of the enamel, in the enamel and outer dentine, or reaching right through the dentine (Figs. 1.18 and 1.19). The pulp is often exposed by the carious process in the latter appearance.

A sharp angled probe (Briault—see Chapter 5) has been recommended to try to determine whether an approximal lesion is cavitated, but if this is done it must be with a gentle touch and not a heavy hand for reasons discussed earlier. If used gently the probe may fall into the cavity if present. Dental floss is less damaging, and if the enamel surface feels rough when floss is passed through the contact point, cavitation is likely to have started.

(a)

(b)

(c)

(d)

Fig. 1.18 The radiographs record the progress of approximal caries on the distal aspect of a mandibular first premolar over a period of 18 months in a patient aged 15–16 years.

(a) Early enamel lesion.

(b) Nine months later—late enamel lesion.

(c) Twelve months later—marked dentinal spread.

(d) Eighteen months later—approaching carious exposure.

Fig. 1.19 Diagrammatic representations of caries on bite-wing radiographs.

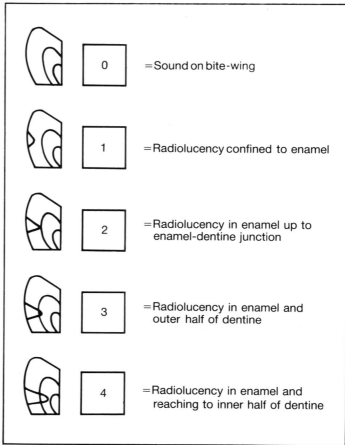

0 = Sound on bite-wing

1 = Radiolucency confined to enamel

2 = Radiolucency in enamel up to enamel-dentine junction

3 = Radiolucency in enamel and outer half of dentine

4 = Radiolucency in enamel and reaching to inner half of dentine

In contrast, an approximal lesion on the root surface may be diagnosed visually if the gingival health is good. If the gingivae are red, swollen, and tend to bleed, detailed caries diagnosis in these areas should be deferred until the teeth have been scaled and cleaned and improved oral hygiene has been achieved.

Caries on the approximal root surface is visible on a bite-wing-radiograph (Fig. 1.20) although its appearance is sometimes confused with the cervical radiolucency. The latter is a perfectly normal appearance at the gap between the dense

Fig. 1.20 A bite-wing radiograph showing root caries on the distal aspect of the upper second premolar, upper first molar, and lower first molar. The arrow points to the cervical radiolucency on the lower third molar. This is a normal appearance but it can sometimes be confused with root caries.

Cervical radiolucency

enamel over the crown of the tooth and the crest of the alveolar ridge where the X-rays pass tangentially through the dentine of the root (not through enamel or bone), giving a relatively radiolucent appearance (Fig. 1.20).

Transmitted light can also be of considerable assistance in the diagnosis of approximal caries, particularly in anterior teeth. The operating light is reflected through the contact point with the dental mirror, and a carious lesion appears as a dark shadow following the outline of the decay (Fig. 1.21).

In posterior teeth (Fig. 1.22) a stronger light source is required, and fibre-optic lights, with the beam reduced to 0.5 mm diameter, have been used. It is important that the diameter of the light source is small so that glare and loss of surface detail are eliminated. The light should be used with dry teeth. The technique has particular advantages in patients with posterior crowding, where bite-wing radiographs will produce overlapping images, and in pregnant women, where unnecessary radiation should be avoided.

Fig. 1.21 A mirror view of the palatal aspect of the upper anterior teeth. A small lesion is visible on the distal aspect of the central incisor and a larger lesion is present on the mesial aspect of the lateral incisor.

Diagnosis of caries on exposed smooth surfaces

Caries on smooth surfaces can be seen at the stage of the white or brown spot lesion before cavitation has occurred, provided that the teeth are clean, dry, and well lit (Fig. 1.5).

Root surface caries, in its early stages, appears as one or more small well-defined discoloured areas located along the gingival margin. Active lesions are soft, whereas arrested or slowly progressing lesions are harder (Fig. 1.23). They are probably softer than the surrounding normal cementum, but often their consistency seems more leathery than that of the active lesion. As with enamel caries, great care should be taken when using a probe on these lesions; otherwise, healing tissue may be damaged. However, it is essential to feel these lesions to determine their activity and an excavator may allow the surface of the lesion to be gently scraped.

Assessment of caries risk

Diagnosis implies more than just recording the number of cavities, their location, and appearance. It is necessary to know whether the patient is likely to develop new cavities and whether existing cavities are likely to progress. Only then can preventive and operative treatment be prescribed which is suitable to the needs of the individual patient.

Figure 1.24 lists some of the many factors relevant to the assessment of caries risk. Social factors will be assessed, often unconsciously, as the patient enters the room. Dress, demeanour, and ethnic background will be apparent for subjective appraisal but must not be allowed to prejudice more objective observations. Questions on employment, attendance patterns, and disease pattern of other family members elicit valuable information. During history taking the patient's dental aspirations become apparent and wise treatment planning will encompass these aspirations. Sadly, dental caries is now principally a problem of the socially deprived, although there are many exceptions.

Medical history is always important in dental practice and some illnesses specifically predispose to a high risk of dental caries. The most important of these are medical problems causing xerostomia, such as radiotherapy in the region of the salivary glands, Sjögren's syndrome, and long-term use of some medications such as tranquillizers, antihypertensives, and diuretics. Frequent medication may itself pose a problem if the medication is sugar-based.

Dietary habits and the patient's attitude to them are of prime importance since diet is one of the main factors in the development of dental caries. For this reason a dietary history is an important part of the assessment in patients with a high caries activity. A diet sheet on which the patient is asked to record everything taken by

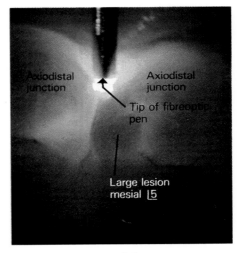

Fig. 1.22 A fibre-optic light in use to assist in the diagnosis of approximal caries. Shadowing indicates a lesion. (Reproduced by courtesy of Dental Update.)

Fig. 1.23 Arrested or slowly progressing root surface caries. This lesion felt hard when an excavator was scraped across it.

FDig. 1.24   Caries risk assessment.

CARIES RISK ASSESSMENT	
HIGH RISK	**LOW RISK**
SOCIAL HISTORY	
Socially deprived High caries in siblings Low knowledge of dental disease Irregular attender Ready availability of snacks Low dental aspirations	Middle class Low caries in siblings Dentally aware Regular attender Work does not allow regular snacks High dental aspirations
MEDICAL HISTORY	
Medically compromised Handicapped Xerostomia Long-term cariogenic medicine	No medical problem No physical problem Normal salivary flow No long-term medication
DIETARY HABITS	
Frequent sugar intake	Infrequent sugar intake
FLUORIDE USE	
Non-fluoride area No fluoride supplements No fluoride toothpaste	Fluoridation area Fluoride supplements used Fluoride toothpaste used
PLAQUE CONTROL	
Infrequent, ineffective, cleaning Poor manual control	Frequent/effective cleaning Good manual control
SALIVA	
Low flow rate Low buffering capacity High *S.mutans* and lactobacillus counts	Normal flow rate Low buffering capacity Low *S.mutans* and lactobacillus counts
CLINICAL EVIDENCE	
New lesions Premature extractions Anterior caries or restorations Multiple restorations History of repeated restorations No fissure sealants Multiband orthodontics Partial dentures	No new lesions Nil extractions for caries Sound anterior teeth No or few restorations Restorations inserted years ago Fissure sealed No appliances

FDig. 1.24   Caries risk assessment.

mouth for a 4 day period, can be a useful record. Figure 1.25 shows such a diet sheet where it seems obvious that frequent sweet drinks, sweets, and other sugar-containing snacks taken before bed are a potential cause of caries in this mouth. Fluoride history is also of importance since the fluoride ion delays lesion progression. It is always wise to check that a fluoride toothpaste is used. It is surprising how often patients with multiple carious lesions select a particular brand of toothpaste, manufactured for sensitive teeth, which does not contain fluoride.

Clinical examination is the most useful indicator of caries risk. A history of repeated restoration and re-restoration, together with multiple new lesions on clinical and/or radiographic examination, is an obvious caries risk. Stagnation areas such as unsealed deep fissures, multiband orthodontic appliances, partial dentures, and poor restorative dentistry encourage plaque accumulation and increase caries risk. Plaque control itself is also relevant, and removal of smooth surface plaque may uncover multiple cervical white spot lesions or cavities in caries-prone mouths.

Diet Analysis

* 2 spoons of sugar

	Thursday		Friday		Saturday		Sunday	
	Time	Item	Time	Item	Time	Item	Time	Item
Before breakfast	7.30	Tea*	7.0	Tea*	7.30	Tea*	7.05	Tea*
Breakfast	8.00	2 Wheat slices 2 Crispbread 1 Apple Coffee*	8.00	2 Wheat slices 2 Crisp bread 1 Apple Coffee*	8.30	2 Wheat slices 2 Crispbread 1 Apple Coffee*	8.05	2 Wheat slices 2 Crispbread 1 Apple Coffee*
Morning	9.00	Polo	10.00 / 11.30	Murray mint / Tea* Biscuit	11.15	Tea*	10.00 / 12.30	Lemon Barley / Tea*
Mid-day Meal	12.30	Meat roll Tea*	2.00	Steamed fish Parsley sauce Boiled potatoes	1.45	Sausage, onion, Boiled potatoes Ice cream, tinned fruit	1.40	Roast lamb, potatoes, cabbage, carrots
Afternoon	2.00 / 5.30	2 Cream crackers 1 Dairy Lea Tea* / 2 Shortbread biscuits Tea*	2.45 / 6.00	Tea* / Tea*	2.30 / 5.45	Tea* / Tea*	2.00 / 4.00	Tea* / Tea*
Evening Meal	8.00	Chop, leeks, boiled potatoes Choc-ice Tea*	8.30	Bacon sandwich Tea*	7.30	Fried kipper bread and butter	8.15	Ham salad, bread and butter Tea*
Evening and night	1.00	Horlicks* Biscuits	10.00 / 1.30	Peanuts / Horlicks* Biscuit	9.15 / 1.45	Chocolate / Horlicks* Biscuits	1.15	Horlicks* Biscuits

Fig. 1.25 A diet sheet completed by a middle-aged patient with a high incidence of caries. The frequent sweet drinks, sweets, and the pre-bed sweet drink and snack are a potential cause of caries in this mouth. Note the frequency of sugar intake—eight times per day.

Fig. 1.26 A proprietary kit used to estimate buffering capacity. The litmus paper is dipped in the patient's saliva and the colour is compared with the manufacturer's chart to read off the patient's buffering capacity. (Reproduced by courtesy of Ivoclar Vivadent Ltd.)

Fig. 1.27 A proprietary kit used to estimate a lactobacillus count. The slide is covered with the patient's saliva and incubated. It is then compared with the manufacturer's chart to estimate the lactobacillus count. (Reproduced by courtesy of Ivoclar Vivadent Ltd.)

Fig. 1.28 A proprietary kit used to estimate a *S. mutans* count. The spatula is rotated on the patient's tongue and incubated in a special culture medium. It is then compared with the manufacturer's chart to estimate the *S. mutans* count. (Reproduced by courtesy of Ivoclar Vivadent Ltd.)

Since saliva is so essential to tooth integrity, its examination is a logical step in caries risk assessment. Stimulated salivary flow rate, buffer capacity, and counts of *Streptococcus mutans* and lactobacilli can all be carried out at the chairside and, in selected patients, such tests may be appropriate. Proprietary kits can be used for these tests. They supply paraffin wax which the patient chews to stimulate saliva. As saliva forms, the patient spits it into a measuring cylinder. A simple litmus type test measures buffering capacity (Fig 1.26) and the saliva can then be poured over a slide which is inoculated with a special medium to allow lactobacilli to grow. The slide is incubated and any lactobacilli in the saliva multiply to form colonies on the slide. The number of colonies can then be estimated by reference to the manufacturer's chart (Fig. 1.27). A similar system is available for estimation of *S. mutans*, although in this case saliva is collected by rotating a special slide on the patient's tongue (Fig 1.28).

It is important to remember that no one factor predisposes to caries risk, but putting all the information together can build up a valuable picture. This enables appropriate preventive strategies to be targeted at high risk patients.

Symptoms of caries

Thus far the signs of caries—that is, what the clinician can detect—have been considered. However, patients often seek treatment for the *symptoms* of caries. What are these symptoms?

Unfortunately, caries presents symptomatically at a relatively late stage. The patient may feel a 'hole in a tooth' with the tongue, brown or black discoloration or cavities may be seen, or frank pain may be suffered.

Caries, even in dentine, is not painful *per se*, but cavitation may occasionally present as mild pain with sweet things or with heat or cold. Normally, the enamel and the necrotic dentine insulate the sensitive dentine and pulp from these stimuli. However, a much more common cause of pain, which may be intense, is pulpitis (the commonest 'toothache') which occurs late in the development of a carious lesion when the caries is very close to the pulp or actually exposing it (see p. 7).

A chronically inflamed pulp may be symptomless or produce only mild symptoms. In contrast, acute pulpitis is very painful, with the pain often being initiated by hot and cold stimuli. Unfortunately, the pain is not well localized to the offending tooth, and the patient may only be able to indicate which quadrant, or even which side, of the mouth is involved. (See Chapter 2 for further details on the diagnosis and management of toothache.)

The relevance of the diagnostic information to the management of caries

There are four approaches to the management of caries:

- attempt to arrest the disease by preventive measures

- remove and replace the carious tissues (operative dentistry)

- a combination of these two approaches

- extract the tooth.

Caries on exposed smooth surfaces

The first time that the patient is seen, it may not be obvious whether small lesions are active or are in a chronic static state which may have been present for many years. Thus, although these lesions are easy to diagnose, it may not be easy to interpret their activity. The wise practitioner will explain the problem to the patient, advocate preventive measures such as dietary advice and improved plaque control, and reassess the lesion in six months. Operative intervention is not required prior to cavitation, and even cavitated lesions can be arrested. Lesions which are plaque traps, unsightly, or deep should be restored.

Caries in pits and fissures

Since this is difficult to diagnose in its early stages and fissures are particularly susceptible sites, the dentist may decide to fissure seal susceptible teeth as soon after eruption as possible. The indications for fissure sealing are given in Chapter 6 (p. 105).

It is also possible to combine fissure sealing with a small restoration in one part of the fissure system. This is called the sealant restoration (p. 108).

The occlusal lesion which shows on a bite-wing radiograph (Fig. 1.17) should be restored. The anatomy of the fissure and the consequent shape of the carious lesion often results in gross undermining of enamel by the carious process, and these lesions are larger than they appear on the radiograph. In addition, the rate of progression of pit and fissure caries may be rapid. In children, the occlusal enamel can be sufficiently undermined to collapse in less than one year from the start of the lesion.

Approximal lesions

These may develop more slowly, taking three to four years to reach dentine in permanent teeth. For this reason, the early nick in outer enamel seen on a bite-wing radiograph (Figs. 1.18a and 1.19) should be given a chance to become arrested by applying preventive measures.

While it is known from clinical studies that the progress of caries through enamel can be slow, the time taken for caries to pass through dentine is unknown although it varies considerably from individual to individual. Caries progressed rapidly in the mouth of the teenagers shown in Figs 1.9 and 1.18.

Once caries is visible in dentine on a bite-wing radiograph, the enamel is likely to be cavitated. Thus, once dentine is involved radiographically, operative treatment is usually indicated. The aim of the treatment is to remove the bacterial infection and restore the integrity of the tooth surface, thus protecting the pulp. Occasionally, however, serial radiographs indicate that even extensive lesions in dentine are static for many years (Fig. 1.29); therefore even this 'rule' should not be applied rigidly.

Root caries

Early diagnosis is of particular clinical importance because advanced disease is extremely difficult to treat by operative means. Lesions may coalesce to encircle the neck of the tooth. It is often possible to reharden such lesions by preventive measures, although as the lesions become arrested, a brownish black discoloration cannot be avoided.

Root caries should be restored where it endangers the pulp, where cavitation is encouraging plaque stagnation, or if sensitivity or appearance are problems.

PREVENTING DENTAL CARIES

Throughout this chapter it has been emphasized that caries is an alternating process of destruction and repair (Fig. 1.30). Since the disease requires plaque bacteria, a carbohydrate substrate, and a susceptible tooth surface, there are three ways of preventing it.

(a)

(b)

Fig. 1.29 An arrested lesion on the distal aspect of the lower second premolar tooth (compare with Fig. 1.18).
(a) Shows the lesion clearly in dentine. Note that caries is also present beneath the occlusal restoration in the lower first molar tooth.
(b) Shows the same lesion in the lower second premolar tooth two years later. Despite the fact that this lesion was not treated operatively, it has not progressed. A new amalgam restoration is present in the lower first molar tooth.

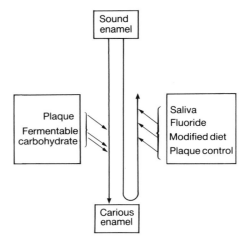

Fig. 1.30 A diagrammatic representation of caries as an alternating process of destruction and repair. Sound enamel will become carious in time if plaque bacteria are given the substrate that they need to produce acid. However, saliva is a remineralizing fluid and the arrows can be turned around towards sound enamel by use of fluoride, by modifying diet, and by attempting to remove plaque.

Fig. 1.31 The most common causes of tooth wear.

Erosion (Most common and most damaging)

Regurgitation erosion

Commonly affects the palatal surfaces of upper anterior teeth and the occlusal and buccal surfaces of lower posterior teeth. Caused by the regurgitation of hydrochloric acid from the stomach in patients with:

- various digestive disorders including hiatus hernia and chronic indigestion.
- anorexia and bulimia nervosa.
- chronic alcoholism.
- morning sickness associated with pregnancy.
- voluntary regurgitation.

Dietary erosion

Commonly affects the labial surfaces of upper anterior teeth. Caused by an excess of food and drink with a low pH including:

- citrus (and other) fruit and fruit juices (citric acid).
- pickles and other food and drink containing vinegar (acetic acid).
- carbonated drinks (carbonic and sometimes other acids).

Industrial erosion

Commonly affects the labial surfaces of the upper anterior teeth and may cause pitting. Caused by industrial processes which produce acid fumes or droplets. Workers should be adequately protected against this and the condition is only rarely seen nowadays.

Attrition

Physical wear of one tooth against another. Affects the incisal edges and occlusal surfaces of opposing teeth. May be accelerated by erosion or may be caused entirely by bruxism or other parafunctional activities.

Abrasion

Commonly affects the neck of the buccal surfaces of both anterior and posterior teeth. The aetiology is not clear, but some dentists believe that it is caused by physical wear from external agents such as:

- abrasive toothpastes and powders (e.g. smokers tooth powder).
- hard toothbrushes or the excessive use of other tooth cleaning aids.
- habits such as thread biting and pipe smoking, can cause wear in the form of notches in the incisal edges

Eliminate the carbohydrate substrate

Fortunately, complete elimination of sugar from the diet is not necessary to prevent caries. Relatively simple measures, such as reducing the frequency of consumption by confining sugar to mealtimes and using a sugar substitute in hot drinks, are usually sufficient.

Increase the resistance of the host

Enamel and exposed dentine can be made more resistant to dental caries by the use of fluoride. Deep pits and fissures can be made more resistant by obliterating or sealing them with a resin fissure sealant (see Chapter 6).

Eliminate bacterial plaque

Theoretically a plaque-free tooth surface will not decay, but complete elimination of plaque is not possible in some areas (e.g. fissures) and not always practical in other areas (e.g. approximally, where plaque elimination requires the skilful use of floss). However, in other areas (e.g. cervically) effective plaque control will prevent caries.

Since this is a textbook of operative dentistry rather than preventive dentistry, these preventive measures will not be discussed further. (See 'Further reading' at the end of this chapter; Kidd and Joyston-Bechal is a simple introduction to preventive dentistry while Thylstrup and Fejerskov is a comprehensive and fully referenced cariology textbook.) However, it is essential that preventive and operative approaches are combined in the management of caries. To do otherwise would be futile and unethical, and could be regarded as negligent. The fact that preventive measures are not always effective, partly because they all require the patient's dedicated co-operation, does not absolve the dentist from making the attempt. Ultimately, it is the patient who will prevent disease, not the dentist, and so a principal responsibility of the profession is to provide patients with enough knowledge to understand their essential role in caries control. They are then in a position to make an informed decision about how they will manage their mouths.

Fig. 1.32 Regurgitation erosion affecting the palatal surfaces of the upper incisor and premolar teeth. This was due, in this case, to bulimia nervosa, sometimes known as 'dietary chaos'. The patients commonly over-eat and then deliberately vomit in an attempt to maintain a low body weight.

TOOTH WEAR

Tooth wear can be defined as the surface loss of dental hard tissues other than by caries or trauma, and is a natural consequence of ageing. It is commonly divided into three components—erosion, attrition, and abrasion—but these conditions often coexist (Fig. 1.31).

Erosion

This is defined as the loss of dental hard tissue as a result of a chemical process not involving bacteria. The causative agent is usually an acid. The source of the acid may be dietary, including foods such as citrus fruits, pickles and other items containing vinegar, or carbonated and acid-containing drinks. Occasionally, acidic medication is implicated.

Alternatively, acid regurgitated from the stomach can cause erosion. This may be associated with anorexia or bulimia nervosa (Fig. 1.32), hiatus hernia, peptic ulcers, pregnancy with prolonged morning sickness or milder forms of digestive disturbance which cause recurrent vomiting, or less severe chronic indigestion (Fig. 1.33). Teeth exposed to industrial acids can also become eroded, although good industrial practice should prevent this. Acid erosion can present as wear on any tooth surface.

Fig. 1.33 Regurgitation erosion. The enamel has lost all its surface characteristics and is very smooth. There is complete loss of enamel at the palatal cervical margins with dentine exposed on all three teeth.

Attrition

This is defined as mechanical wear between opposing teeth (Fig. 1.34) and commonly occurs in combination with erosion. By definition, attrition presents on contacting occlusal or incisal surfaces, but where erosion and attrition coexist, some areas of the worn occlusal surface may not contact in any mandibular excursion. This pattern shows that attrition cannot be entirely responsible for the tooth wear and that an erosive element must also be present (Fig. 1.35). The physical effect of food wearing the tooth surface is not well understood, but it is thought to have little effect in contemporary diets in Western countries. It may be of more relevance in particularly abrasive diets (e.g. some vegetarians).

Fig. 1.34 Attrition. The patient is making a right lateral excursion of the mandible and the upper and lower teeth fit well together at this point. It is likely that the patient bruxes in this position at night. Note also that the upper and lower teeth are worn by approximately the same amount.

Fig. 1.35 Incisal wear which is the result of a combination of erosion and attrition. The incisal edges are cupped out and do not make contact with the opposing teeth in any excursion of the mandible.

Fig. 1.34   Fig. 1.35

Abrasion

This is the wearing away of tooth substance by mechanical means other than by opposing teeth, such as holding a pipe or perhaps over-vigorous tooth-brushing. It is easy to understand how tooth tissue softened by acid is particularly susceptible to such wear, and it can be difficult to make a clear distinction between erosion and abrasion. Abrasion-erosion lesions commonly present buccally at the cervical margin, and are either dish-shaped or in the form of a sharp V-shaped notch (Fig. 1.36). The reason for these two distinctly different presentations is not known.

Fig. 1.36 (a) Dish-shaped abrasion–erosion lesions. Large areas of dentine are exposed at the base of saucer-shaped lesions. (b) V-shaped notch lesions which occur at the necks of teeth. Note also that all the enamel surfaces have been worn smooth.

(a)   **(b)**

Acceptable and pathological levels of tooth wear

It is normal for teeth to wear, but the process is regarded as pathological if they become so worn that they function ineffectively or seriously mar appearance. The distinction between acceptable and pathological tooth wear at a given age is based on a prediction as to whether the tooth will survive that rate of wear in a functional and reasonably aesthetic state until the end of the patient's normal lifespan.

Consequences of pathological tooth wear

There are several important clinical features that can result from pathological tooth wear. These include the following:

- exposure of dentine on buccal or lingual surfaces normally covered by enamel (Fig. 1.33)

- notched cervical surfaces (Fig. 1.36)

- exposure of dentine on incisal or occlusal surfaces—further erosion often results in preferential loss of dentine to produce a cupped surface (Fig. 1.35)

- restorations (which do not erode) left projecting above the tooth surface

- exposure of reparative dentine or pulp

- wear producing sensitivity

- pulpitis and loss of vitality attributable to tooth wear

- wear in one arch more than in the other

- inability to make contact between worn incisal or occlusal surfaces in any excursion of the mandible

- reduction in length of the incisor teeth so that length is out of proportion to width.

Some of these features require operative intervention to protect the pulp, reduce sensitivity, and improve appearance or function. However, restorations will not prevent further wear. Just as with dental caries, restoration can temporarily replace the lost tooth surface but wear will continue on any tooth surface exposed around the restoration if the cause is not identified and prevented.

Diagnosing and monitoring tooth wear

It is relatively easy to diagnose that teeth are worn, provided that they are viewed clean and dry. Differentiating between acceptable and pathological levels of wear can be more difficult because the decision depends on the age of the patient. Also, a single examination will not show whether the wear is static or progressing, nor the speed of any progression.

Where a pathological rate of tooth wear is suspected, study models taken at six-monthly or yearly intervals will determine the rate of progress and the effectiveness of preventive measures. If these measures are not entirely successful, the series of models will help to decide if and when to intervene operatively.

Assessing the aetiology

Finding the cause of tooth wear can be very difficult, but a careful sympathetic history is helpful. Many of these patients have conditions which they find difficult or embarrassing to discuss, such as bulimia nervosa, anorexia nervosa, or chronic alcoholism. Bulimia nervosa is a variation of anorexia nervosa in which the patient deliberately vomits repeatedly (often between 2 and 30 times a day) in an attempt to control body weight. Eating habits are bizarre and compulsive, and the patients tend to be secretive about them and do not regard themselves as ill. The repeated vomiting often causes very rapid erosion, occasionally so fast that vital pulps are exposed.

Chronic alcoholism causes a chronic gastritis which in turn produces dental erosion in some patients even without recurrent frank vomiting.

The history might include questions on the following topics.

Relating to erosion

- Past and present diet, including questions on a series of food and drink items known to cause dietary erosion (Fig. 1.31).

- Digestive disorders which may produce a regurgitation erosion, including pregnancy sickness.

- Past and present slimming habits, including any tendency to anorexic or bulimic behaviour.

- Weight loss that might be indicative of anorexia.

- Alcohol intake.

- Past and present medical history and medication, including vitamin C, iron preparations, and hydrochloric acid for achlorhydria.

- The patient's present and past occupation relevant to industrial erosion.

Figure 1.37 provides a useful *aide-mémoire* for the inexperienced clinician who finds the variety and complexity of the questions a lot to remember.

Relating to attrition

- Clenching and grinding habits. Has a sleeping partner heard grinding noises?

- Periods of stress or anxiety.

- Other habits including pipe smoking, opening hairgrips, and biting thread.

- Has the patient a 'square jaw' with over-developed muscles?

Relating to abrasion

- Oral hygiene techniques, including past and present use of abrasive tooth-cleaning techniques and materials.

- Habits which might abrade teeth such as pipe smoking.

On the basis of the answers to these questions it may be possible to define the aetiology as one of the following:

- dietary erosion

- regurgitation erosion

- industrial erosion

- attrition

- abrasion

- combined aetiology (try to assess the importance of each aetiological factor)

- aetiology not determined.

A study of the causes of tooth wear showed that dietary and regurgitation erosion were the most common, with regurgitation erosion causing the most severe damage. Of a group of 100 patients with severe tooth wear, a definite diagnosis could not be made in 30 of them, thus emphasizing the difficulty of reliably assessing the true cause of this problem.

Preventing tooth wear

Prevention clearly depends primarily on making an accurate diagnosis of the cause. Some erosive causes, once identified, are easy to prevent; others are more difficult. For example, a patient with an erosive dietary fad, such as sucking lemons, may be willing to forgo the habit, but chronic alcoholics are much less likely to change for the sake of their teeth alone.

Attrition due to nocturnal bruxism may be helped by occlusal adjustment to remove interferences which trigger the grinding, and in other cases an acrylic bite

Name...   Number... Sex   M   F
Address ....   Tel No ....
     ....   Occupation ....
     ....   Work Place ....

Interests, hobbies, sport activities ....
Medication ....
Illness Present .... Illness past ....
Has the illness been treated .... By a doctor .... In hospital ....

GASTRIC SYMPTOMS	PAST SYMPTOMS			NO	PRESENT SYMPTOMS		
	Frequency per week	Frequency per day	Duration		Frequency per week	Frequency per day	Duration
Belching							
Heart burn							
Acid taste in the mouth							
Vomiting							
Regurgitation ? chew cud							
Stomach ache							
Gastric pain on awakening							
How does the patient treat gastric pain?							
DIET	PAST CONSUMPTION			NO	PRESENT CONSUMPTION		
	Frequency per week	Frequency per day	Duration		Frequency per week	Frequency per day	Duration
Citrus fruits							
Citrus fruit juice							
Other juices							
Special juices							
Sport drinks							
Fruit berries							
Soft drinks, acidic beverages							
Yoghurt							
Vitamin-C drinks, chewable tablets							
Acid sweets							
Special diet							
Vinegar							
Herb tea							
Pickles							
Other acidic food etc							
Alcohol							

Fig. 1.37 An *aide-mémoire* for use when taking a history relating to erosion.

plane is provided for use at nights. This may reduce the grinding habit and will absorb the wear, with the acrylic being replaced periodically.

Abrasion may be prevented by changing the abrasive activity, for instance the method of tooth-brushing and/or the toothpaste used.

The management of tooth wear

Unlike caries, tooth wear is an irreversible process. Management should have the objective of maintaining a functional comfortable dentition of good appearance for life, so the emphasis should be on prevention and monitoring in the early stages, avoiding the temptation of placing restorations until they are necessary. They become necessary only when the patient becomes concerned about the appearance, or the teeth become sensitive, or the dentist becomes concerned about physical changes such as changes in occlusal vertical dimension or pulp exposure. If restorations are placed while the wear is progressing, particularly in erosion, they may accelerate rather than slow down the rate of wear in the surrounding tooth tissue. In advanced cases, crowns are required.

TRAUMA

While caries and tooth wear are diseases of slow onset, traumatic injuries are acquired suddenly, and when these involve the hard dental tissues and the pulp they usually require immediate operative management. Trauma to the mouth can produce these local injuries:

- lacerations to the lips, tongue, and gingival tissue

- alveolar fractures, so that a number of teeth become mobile within a block of bone

- complete or partial subluxation of a tooth

- root fracture

- damage to the apical blood vessels without fracture

- fracture of the crown of the tooth involving enamel alone, enamel and dentine, or exposure of the pulp.

These injuries can, of course, occur in combination. Only the last one listed will be discussed in detail here.

Aetiology of trauma

Trauma is commonly caused by the following:

- falls

- sports or athletics

- blows from foreign bodies

- fights

- car or bicycle accidents

- injuries during convulsive seizures (e.g. epilepsy)

- battered child syndrome (the most difficult and yet the most important to diagnose).

Examination and diagnosis of dental injury

When other injuries have also been sustained, particularly head injuries, these must be investigated and dealt with before detailed examination and treatment of the dental injury. When this has been done a careful history of the accident as it relates to the teeth must be recorded, together with any symptoms such as pain, fracture, or loosening of teeth.

An examination must be made for any extra-oral wounds and injuries to the mucosa and the gingivae. The crowns of the teeth are examined for fractures, pulp exposure, and colour changes. Displacement or looseness of teeth should be noted, together with abnormalities of the occlusion.

The vitality of the injured and adjacent (and usually the opposing) teeth must be tested (see Chapter 2) and periapical radiographs must always be taken to look for root fracture. Where fractures of the maxilla or mandible are suspected, further radiographs of the facial skeleton will be required. Where teeth are fractured and the inside of the lips is lacerated, radiographs should be taken of the soft tissues to check that fragments of teeth are not present.

At subsequent recall visits the colour of the tooth and further vitality tests and periapical radiographs will show whether the pulp has remained vital or not. If the tooth begins to discolour (Fig. 1.38), this is a sign that the pulp has died and it should be removed immediately to prevent the risk of acute infection and further discoloration.

Fig. 1.38 A discoloured upper right central incisor resulting from a necrotic untreated pulp.

Management of trauma to the teeth

Where enamel is crazed or slightly chipped either no treatment or simply smoothing the enamel may be all that is required. However, the vitality of such teeth should be checked periodically and new periapical radiographs taken to look for signs of pulp death.

Where fracture of enamel and dentine has occurred (Fig. 1.39) the exposed dentine is often very sensitive to hot, cold, and sweet stimuli, and the patient's appearance may be affected. Usually, a tooth-coloured composite restoration is required at once (with a suitable lining to protect the pulp) to restore appearance (see Chapter 9). Again, the tooth must be checked for vitality and periapical radiographs taken periodically.

Where the fracture has exposed the pulp it is often necessary to remove the pulp tissue, as pulp necrosis is likely to occur. In young teeth with incompletely formed apices only the coronal pulp tissue is removed (pulpotomy) and a calcium hydroxide dressing is placed on the remaining pulpal tissue so that the apex can continue to form. The crown of the tooth is restored with tooth-coloured composite and subsequently a root canal filling is placed.

Teeth which have become discoloured following trauma can be bleached after root filling (see Chapter 9). If this is not successful, the buccal surface can be veneered with composite (see Chapter 9) or porcelain (see Chapter 10), or a crown can be made.

The management of root fractures, tooth extrusions, avulsions, and intrusions is beyond the scope of this book.

Fig. 1.39 A fractured incisor involving enamel and dentine, but not the pulp. (By courtesy of Mr P. Longhurst.)

DEVELOPMENTAL DEFECTS

Teeth do not always develop normally, and there are a number of defects in tooth structure or shape which occur during development and become apparent on eruption. Such teeth are often unsightly or prone to excessive tooth wear, and thus they may require restoration to improve appearance or function or to protect the underlying tooth structure.

Acquired developmental conditions

Enamel hypoplasia and hypomineralization

Fig. 1.40 Hypoplastic enamel in a patient who had a severe childhood illness. The pitted enamel is symmetrically distributed and occurs at the point on the tooth which was developing at the time of the illness.

Ameloblasts are specialized cells that are vulnerable to the effects of generalized systemic conditions such as the infectious diseases of childhood. Alternatively, they may be damaged by adverse local conditions such as trauma to or infection of a deciduous predecessor.

The usual consequence of damage to the ameloblasts is the formation of either hypoplastic or hypomineralized enamel.

Hypoplastic enamel results from the production of a reduced amount of matrix which matures normally; thus, the enamel is pitted or thin but of normal hardness (Fig. 1.40).

Hypomineralized enamel results when a normal amount of matrix fails to achieve full mineralization. The affected enamel has a normal shape and thickness but has an opaque chalky white appearance (Fig. 1.41).

The degree of hypoplasia or hypomineralization that results from a systemic disturbance reflects its severity, timing, and duration. Consequently, systemic disturbances usually affect multiple teeth, and the position of the enamel defect corresponds to the enamel formed at the time of the disturbance. The majority of systemic disturbances last only a few weeks and for this reason the defect takes the form of a narrow horizontal band around the affected crown or crowns. Since all the developing crowns are affected, the resulting lesions are bilaterally symmetrical (Fig. 1.40).

Fig. 1.41 Hypomineralized enamel.

Generalized intrinsic enamel stain

Two substances which may be ingested during tooth formation are of particular importance; these are the fluoride ion and the drug tetracycline.

Dental fluorosis

Dental fluorosis may occur when the total daily intake of the fluoride ion from sources such as water, toothpaste, drops, and tablets is high. It may be seen as a number of chalky white flecks or confluent blotches and brown discoloration sometimes accompanied by pitting of the enamel (Fig. 1.42). Most severe cases are seen in areas where the fluoride content of the natural water supply is high, such as parts of Africa and India.

Fig. 1.42 Enamel fluorosis resulting in white mottling of all the teeth and brown discoloration of the upper incisor teeth.

Tetracycline staining

Tetracycline staining is a cause of tooth discoloration which should never happen. This group of broad spectrum antibiotics has an affinity for calcified tissue. It can cross the placental barrier to affect the deciduous teeth. If the drug is taken by infants and young children the developing permanent teeth will usually be discoloured (Fig. 1.43). If tetracycline staining is to be avoided, this group of drugs should not be administered in pregnancy or to children under 12 years.

Treatment of acquired developmental conditions

Because these conditions do not progress, the treatment can be deferred until the patient is concerned about the appearance. The aim of treatment is almost entirely cosmetic, but no less important for that.

Bleaching may be effective in some cases of tetracycline stain, but in most cases composite restorations or veneers of composite or porcelain, often with little or no tooth preparation, are the treatment of choice. Crowns may be necessary in the most severe cases.

Fig. 1.43 Severe tetracycline stain. Note the horizontal banding which does not appear to be related to the stage of development of the tooth at which the drug was administered.

Hereditary conditions

The inherited conditions which may result in defects in tooth number, shape, size, or structure are hypodontia, microdontia, amelogenesis imperfecta, and dentinogenesis imperfecta. Fortunately the two last conditions are rare.

Hypodontia, microdontia

Hypodontia (sometimes known as oligodontia) is a condition, usually with a strong family history, in which some teeth do not form at all. It may be associated with microdontia, where some teeth are abnormal in shape or size (Fig. 1.44). However, the enamel is normal in texture and colour. Third molars, upper and lower second premolars, and upper lateral incisor teeth are the most commonly affected. Of the three, the upper lateral incisor teeth, and other incisors and canines where they are affected, are the most important to the operative dentist. In hypodontia it may be necessary to alter the shape of adjacent teeth by restorations or crowns, with or without preparatory orthodontic treatment, to improve the patient's appearance. In microdontia it is often possible to alter the shape of the affected teeth.

Fig. 1.44 Microdontia of the upper right lateral incisor (a peg-shaped lateral). The upper left lateral incisor tooth is missing (hypodontia).

Amelogenesis imperfecta

This is a condition associated with extensive abnormalities of enamel formation. At least two different clinical patterns are recognized.

Generalized hypoplasia of the enamel involves a defect of matrix formation, although the matrix present appears normally mineralized. In its severe form the defect results in thin enamel with teeth appearing yellow because the underlying dentine shows through. A less severe form of the defect presents as a granular or pitted enamel surface which may pick up stain (Fig. 1.45).

In contrast, *generalized hypomineralization* of the enamel involves a normal amount of matrix formation, but its subsequent maturation is faulty and incomplete. The quantity of the enamel is normal but the tissue is frequently soft, friable, and easily lost. This enamel may appear stained and darkened or dull and chalky white.

Fig. 1.45 Amelogenesis imperfecta. Not only is the enamel deeply pitted and stained in this 16-year-old girl but there is considerable gingival inflammation resulting from very poor oral hygiene. There are two reasons for the poor oral hygiene: the pitted teeth are very difficult to clean, but, perhaps more importantly, because the patient was so unhappy about her dental appearance it was very difficult to persuade her to take trouble over cleaning them. Nevertheless crowns were provided and her appearance and oral hygiene both improved dramatically.

Dentinogenesis imperfecta

There is deficient formation of dentine and the condition is characterized by an opalescent discoloration of the teeth, which are prone to early fracture and excessive wear (Fig.1.46). Radiographs typically show pulpal obliteration and shortened roots with small bulbous crowns. The treatment of this condition is beyond the scope of this book.

Fig. 1.46 Dentinogenesis imperfecta.

FURTHER READING

Andreasen, J. O. and Andreasen, F. M. (1990). *Essentials of traumatic injuries to the teeth*. Munksgaard, Copenhagen.

Kidd, E. A. M. and Joyston-Bechal, S. (1996). *Essentials of dental caries*. Oxford Medical Publications, Oxford.

Kidd, E. A. M. and Smith, B. G. N. (1993). Toothwear histories: a sensitive issue. *Dent. Update.* **20**, 174–8.

Smith, B. G. N. (1991). Some facets of tooth wear. *Ann. R. Aust. Coll. Dent. Surg.* **11**, 37–51.

Smith, B. G. N. and Knight, J. K. (1984). An index for measuring the wear of teeth. *Br. Dent. J.* **156**, 435–8.

Smith, B. G. N. and Knight, J. K. (1984). A comparison of patterns of tooth wear. *Br. Dent. J.* **157**, 16–19.

Thylstrup, A. and Fejerskov, O. (1994). *Textbook of clinical cariology*. Munksgaard, Copenhagen.

Winter, G. B. and Rapp, R. (1979). *A colour atlas of clinical conditions in paedodontics*, pp. 147–94. Wolfe Medical Publications, London.

2 Making clinical decisions

WHO MAKES THE DECISIONS?

Gone are the days when most patients attended their dentist or other professional adviser, sought and accepted his or her advice without question, and felt almost detached from the process. Although patients used to do things 'under doctor's orders', many now take a much more lively interest in the management of their own health. Indeed, without this involvement by the patient, the preventive measures described in Chapter 1 would be impossible. Along with this involvement, which many patients seek and which should be encouraged in those who do not, comes a responsibility for participating in decisions about their own welfare. In the final analysis, it is patients who will decide whether they will attend for treatment, whether they will clean their teeth effectively, and what sacrifices of time, effort, and finance they are prepared to make.

A dentist's role is to offer advice and, if the advice is accepted, provide treatment. This advice can usually be classified as follows:

- diagnosis

- prognosis

- treatment options

- prevention of further disease.

These matters will be dealt with in more detail shortly, but first it is necessary to understand the nature and status of this professional advice.

Professionalism

The professional-client relationship is special in that professional people take upon themselves the duty of setting their clients' interests above their own. It is this aspect of professionalism which engenders trust in patients and explains why they so often accept the advice of the dentist. Once this professional relationship begins to break down, as it does if the dentist puts his/her own interests before that of the patient, then the patient's confidence is lost and he/she begins to mistrust the dentist's advice. This is quite different from the shared involvement in the management of a condition such as dental caries or tooth wear as described in Chapter 1.

In order to give advice the dentist will need information, and a large part of this chapter is taken up with describing what this information might be, and how it should be collected and collated. In some cases this information alone will be enough to enable the dentist to give advice and take a decision. However, in many cases another element, *judgement*, will need to be applied. If all diagnosis and treatment planning were straightforward, so that a given set of facts always resulted in the same treatment plan, the process could, and by now probably would, be undertaken by computers. Judgement based on the clinician's own experience and that of others is a second element in the essential nature of a professional person. Using the terminology of British law, some of these judgements can be made 'beyond reasonable doubt' but others have to be made 'on the balance of probability'. It is the skill and care with which these judgements are made that distinguishes the really good dentist from the merely good dentist. In difficult cases many experienced clinicians seek second or even third opinions, discussing the case with colleagues before reaching a final decision as to the best advice to offer the patient.

Large and small decisions

Many decisions are rather routine in their nature and become automatic with practice, rather like the subconscious decision to press the accelerator to drive the car faster. While learning to drive, this decision, like many similar decisions in dentistry, has to be considered consciously. Other decisions may be slightly more difficult, such as whether all the dentine caries in a tooth must be removed and whether fissure caries has extended to the point where it should be restored or not (see Chapters 1 and 6); these decisions are always made at the conscious level. Then there are the much more substantial decisions which sometimes have to be made— for example, whether to advise a patient to have all his or her teeth extracted, or to have them all crowned or extensively restored, or to adopt some middle course of a few extractions with a simpler level of restorations and perhaps a partial denture.

THE FOUR MAIN DECISIONS

Diagnosis

Diagnosis is the recognition of a disease. Sometimes a bald statement of the diagnosis is sufficient; for example, amelogenesis imperfecta. In most cases, however, the diagnosis should include the extent, location, and other characteristics of the disease. For example, a diagnosis of caries or periodontal disease is not enough without describing where it occurs and how extensive it is.

Techniques for diagnosing dental caries, tooth wear, tooth trauma, and developmental defects were described in Chapter 1.

Prognosis

The prognosis of a condition is the estimate of what will happen if it is not treated and what the consequences of treatment will be. Therefore the prognosis for an early enamel carious lesion is good if appropriate preventive measures are taken, whereas the prognosis for maintaining the vitality of the pulp if caries is so extensive that symptoms of pulpitis arise is poor. However, in the latter case, if other conditions are favourable, the prognosis for keeping the tooth if root canal treatment is carried out is good.

Treatment options

This often seems to be the most important decision, particularly for the patient, in that it affects what will be done. However, it is based so fundamentally on the first two decisions, diagnosis and prognosis, that it is, in reality, no more important, and often less so, than they are. Chapters 6–11 clarify the options available in given situations together with the reasons for choosing between them.

Further preventive measures

As was shown in Chapter 1, the long-term success of treatment is dependent in many cases on the patient's willingness and ability to co-operate in preventing further disease. A decision about the likelihood of this being effective should be attempted before the definitive treatment plan is decided, in particular if extensive treatment is contemplated. Thus the aim of an initial treatment plan may be to stabilize active disease, assess its cause, and start preventive measures. The patient's response to this initial treatment will be an important factor when planning subsequent care.

THE INFORMATION NEEDED TO MAKE DECISIONS AND HOW IT IS COLLECTED AND RECORDED

Part of the skill of an experienced clinician is to decide what information is needed, and to acquire it accurately and rapidly so that he or she is in the best position to give good advice without undue delay. Some clinicians adopt a 'data gathering' approach in which, using check-lists, they try to accumulate all the information which would conceivably be of some relevance about a patient. To do this comprehensively requires several hours of discussion and examination, and this is clearly impractical and unnecessary in most cases. An example of a questionnaire used to gather information about a patient with dental erosion was shown in Fig. 1.37. Some clinicians find this systematic approach useful, and it is particularly valuable to the inexperienced. Others find that a more discursive approach helps the patient to open up and discuss matters which are sometimes embarrassing or difficult to talk about. These two approaches, which are not mutually exclusive and thus may be combined, are discussed in Kidd and Smith (1993) referred to at the end of Chapter 1.

Some information is essential for all patients, some is useful for most, and in others a very detailed investigation of a narrow field of interest is necesssary in order to reach a diagnosis or make one of the other decisions outlined above. Figure 2.1 shows a list of information which may be helpful to a student when first meeting patients. It is not meant to be followed slavishly but it is a useful *aide-mémoire* for the inexperienced.

However, it is dangerous to begin the examination of a patient without first ensuring that it will pose no risk to either the patient or the dentist. For this reason a full medical history should be taken before the examination, irrespective of any other history.

Lists such as the one in Fig. 2.1 are an oversimplification and suggest that the entire history should be taken first, followed by the examination of the patient. Some dentists even do this in two separate areas of the surgery, attempting to separate the conversational and clinical aspects of the process. This is often not practical and indeed may be undesirable. It is much better to mix the two processes together and maintain a steady conversation with the patient before, during, and after the examination, pausing to take notes or, better still, dictating them to the dental nurse or onto a tape as the process continues.

The reason for this is that until the dentist has made an initial examination of the mouth it is often not possible to tell what detailed line of questioning to pursue. For example, if the patient complains of discoloured teeth, a quick examination will show whether this is surface or intrinsic stain. If it is surface stain there is no need for questioning on the administration of tetracycline in childhood or the ingestion of excessive fluoride. Another common example is the patient who complains about his teeth 'crumbling away'. This may be the result of caries and failing restorations,

History

C/O
HPC
Commencement
Location
Type
Incidence
Duration
Initiating factors
Relieving factors

PDH
Current treatment
Regularity of visits
Treatment received
Ortho
Perio
Cons
Surgical and why
Prosth
Advice on prevention
?Fluoride

GMH
Rheumatic fever
Heart disease
Chest disease
Jaundice or hepatitis
Medication and drugs
Allergies
Abnormal bleeding
Hospital admissions
Operations
Other serious illnesses
Abnormal reaction to
anaesthetic
Pregnancy
Contact with HIV or AIDS

SH
Work
Time to travel
Availability for treatment

HABITS
OH
Diet
Smoking
Alcohol
Bruxing, clenching

Examination

Extra-oral
Symmetry
Lips
Nodes
TMJ

Intraoral

Mucosa
cheeks
palate
tongue
floor of mouth
edentulous ridges
sulci

Periodontium
gingivae
oral hygiene
calculus
pockets
mobility
periodontal charts

Teeth
overall assessment,
caries, tooth wear and
restoration status.
comments specific to
one tooth
caries chart

Occlusion
intercuspal position
retruded contact position
lateral excursions
protrusion
fremitus
faceting

Prosthesis
type, material, support
teeth replaced
appearance
tooth wear
retention, stability

Special tests

Vitality
Radiographs
Study models
Diet analysis

KEY

C/O	Complaining of
HPC	History of present complaint
PDH	Past dental history
GMH	General medical history
SH	Social history

Fig. 2.1 *Aide-mémoire* for the history and examination of the new patient.

tooth wear, or a developmental defect. Again, a quick examination will show which approach to the dietary history is likely to be most helpful—to pursue a detailed history relating to sugar or a detailed history relating to erosive materials—or whether, if it is a developmental disturbance, diet has no bearing on the matter at all. It is necessary here to describe the history and examination process in some sort of order, even if this order will seldom be followed comprehensively in practice. An example of a typical sequence of events mixing the aspects of the history and examination into an order for a given patient is given on p. 39.

History

The following information is usually needed.

About the patient

Name, address, telephone and Fax numbers
This information is essential and it should always be checked for accuracy. It is quite possible to have two people with the same name in the waiting room or the practice, and only careful and routine checking will prevent serious mistakes being made.

Age, sex, occupation
Age will have considerable bearing on the state of dental development in younger patients and is important for a variety of reasons at other ages. The patient's sex usually has no bearing on the treatment advised, although it is usually recorded to avoid confusion. It should not be assumed that female patients are more concerned with their appearance than male patients. The patient's occupation may have a bearing on the condition itself (for example, industrial erosion) and may affect availability for treatment.

Attitude and motivation to dental health and treatment
Whereas information about age and occupation are easily obtained by direct questioning, assessment of attitude to dental health and motivation is more difficult. Direct questioning is usually unhelpful because the patient will tend to answer the questions in a way which will 'please' the dentist. However, attitudes may become apparent during conversation, particularly when past dental treatment and experience are discussed.

Diet
Since diet plays a major role in dental caries and can be of importance in tooth wear, a discussion about diet is often useful. A question such as 'Do you think you have a sweet or a sour tooth?' can often elicit valuable information about attitudes as well as facts. For instance, the way that the patient answers such questions may reveal whether he or she appreciates the relevance of diet to dental disease and whether modification of diet has been tried in the past. However, a detailed examination of diet is reserved for those with specific caries or tooth wear problems which will only become obvious after clinical examination. This is an example of how history and clinical examination go together to produce information relevant to the *particular patient*.

Habits
It is useful to enquire about tooth cleaning habits and the toothpaste used, but other habits may also be relevant; for example, smoking will increase the likelihood of surface stain on teeth. Following clinical examination further questions may be needed; for example, a particular pattern of tooth wear may suggest questions about grinding habits, an erosive diet, or alcohol consumption.

Any apparent discrepancy between what patients say that they do when they clean their teeth and the clinical condition may be cleared up by asking them to bring brush and paste to the surgery.

Willingess to meet fees and other expenses
Most dental treatment involves the patient in some expense. This will be the full professional fee in some cases, while in third-party payment schemes (e.g. the UK National Health Service) there is often a partial fee to be paid. Even in 'free' systems (e.g. treatment by students in UK Dental Schools) the patient may have to take time off work and lose income. Usually, it is not possible to estimate the fee or the amount of time involved until an outline treatment plan is established. Sometimes this 'ideal' outline plan will be too costly for the patient and an alternative might have to be sought. It is important to establish this at an early stage before too much time is spent in detailed planning.

About the patient's general condition and health

Here a check-list is useful and questions are usually asked, and followed up when necessary, about the following:

- history of heart or chest disease

- current (or recent) medication

- allergies

- any difficulty in the arrest of haemorrhage after extraction or injury

- previous hospital admissions

- other diseases

- pregnancy

- contact with HIV or AIDS

When these questions are answered positively it may be necessary to refer to the patient's general medical practitioner or to arrange further investigations (for example, blood tests) before proceeding with treatment.

The patient's reason for attendance

Some patients have an urgent problem such as pain or trauma, while others attend for a routine examination without particular symptoms. When symptoms are present the patient should be encouraged (without the use of leading questions) to describe these as clearly and in as much detail as possible. Some indication of the relevance of painful symptoms was given in Chapter 1 and will be expanded under the heading 'Diagnosing toothache' on p. 42.

Past dental history

A patient's past dental history can be of considerable assistance. Previous treatment indicates susceptibility to disease as well as attitudes towards dental care. For instance, the question 'Have you had many fillings done?' may lead the patient to explain that most teeth have been restored. If this question is then followed up by asking whether most of the fillings are old or whether they have to be replaced regularly, the information obtained may indicate whether the patient is currently a high caries risk. It is thus possible to build up a picture of past dental history which may include caries experience, restorative treatment received, susceptibility to periodontal disease, periodontal treatment received, extractions and the reason for the loss of the teeth, and information about prosthetic replacements.

Family and social background

Where an inherited condition is suspected, clearly the distribution within the family is important. In other cases attitudes to dental health, either positive or negative, engendered within the family may have an important bearing on the condition with which the patient presents or upon acceptance of treatment. The same is true of the patient's social background. Other aspects of the social history—for example, availability for long appointments—will also determine the type of treatment.

Examination

General appearance

The patient may appear nervous or relaxed, fit and well or elderly or ill, clean and tidy or dirty and dishevelled. These or similar observations will guide but should not dictate treatment. It takes time to get to know people and instant judgements are unwise. For instance, a neglected general appearance does not necessarily mean that the person does not care about his dental health.

Factors which predispose to cross-infection
Some people—for example, drug addicts, homosexuals, or heavily tattooed patients—are more likely to be carriers of the hepatitis B virus and HIV (human immunodeficiency virus).

The extra-oral facial appearance

The temporomandibular joint and lymph nodes should be palpated. Any obvious asymmetry is noted and the lips are examined. Such things as injuries or scars on the lips may be accompanied by dental injuries. Where the patient's problem involves appearance, the dentist will make his or her own assessment of this while listening to the patient.

The mouth in general

Oral hygiene is relevant in both periodontal disease and caries. A general impression of whether the mouth is well cared for by both the patient and previous dentists is useful, but patients do sometimes increase their dental awareness considerably and previous neglect need not imply future neglect (Fig. 2.2).

Specific areas of the mouth

The soft tissues
A routine examination of the inner aspects of the lip, the tongue, and the buccal and lingual sulci should be made at *all* examinations since, amongst other things, early neoplastic change can be detected and early treatment can be life-saving (Fig. 2.3).

The periodontal tissues
A general assessment of the state of periodontal health is always necessary. This will include oral hygiene; the presence of both supra- and subgingival calculus, the health and position of the gingival tissues, the presence of pockets, and whether there is bleeding on probing and mobility of teeth. In many cases a more detailed periodontal examination (see later) needs to be undertaken.

Caries experience past and present
Again, a general impression can be gained of the extent of carious lesions and previous restorations. It is reasonable to assume that restorations are most commonly the result of caries but, of course, other conditions (see Chapter 1) may also have been responsible.

(a)

(b)

Fig. 2.2   (a) Before and (b) after a course of treatment by an undergraduate dental student. This patient presented with a very neglected mouth and with poor motivation and low expectations of treatment. However, he not only benefited from the student's treatment but also heeded the advice and encouragement given. He is now highly motivated towards maintaining his remaining teeth and his whole attitude to dentistry has been changed by this experience.

Fig. 2.3   Early neoplastic change in the lower lip. The lip was hard and a biopsy showed squamous cell carcinoma. Without careful observations this lesion could have been mistaken for other less serious conditions. (Courtesy of Dr P. R. Morgan.)

Other conditions affecting the teeth
These include trauma, tooth wear, dental defects, missing teeth, and malpositioned teeth.

The general state of the restorations
See Chapter 11.

The occlusion
First, the static relationship of the teeth in *intercuspal position* (ICP) should be examined to determine the horizontal and vertical overlap of the anterior teeth (overjet and overbite), together with the relationship of the posterior teeth. Next, and perhaps more importantly, the way in which the teeth function against each other in forwards, backwards, and lateral movements of the mandible should be examined. This is often relevant to the decision as to how to restore a tooth. If a cusp functions vigorously against an opposing tooth when the jaw moves, then it may need protecting in some way by the restoration, but if it immediately discludes in all movements of the mandible, it may not (Fig. 2.4).

Fig. 2.4 The patient is making a left lateral excursion of the mandible. The buccal cusp of the upper first premolar is not in contact with the opposing teeth, but the buccal cusps of the upper second premolar and first molar teeth are in contact. Therefore these cusps are at greater risk if they are weakened by caries undermining them than in the case of the upper first premolar tooth.

Dentures
The presence and nature of dentures should be noted. It is important to decide whether dentures are satisfactory or in need of replacement. If abutment teeth for satisfactory dentures need to be restored, a decision must be made as to whether these teeth can be restored to fit the denture and, if so, how this can be done. Alternatively, if new dentures are necessary, they must be designed before planning any restorations required in the abutment teeth. This is important because design features relevant to the dentures (for example, guide planes, rest seats, undercuts for clasps) should be incorporated into the abutment restoration.

Detailed charts

In some cases much more detailed information is required.

Periodontal charting
This may include plaque indices, probing depths, bleeding points, gingival level, and tooth mobility.

Conservation charting
This will include caries and existing restorations. The recognition of caries was described in some detail in Chapter 1 and so it is only necessary here to describe how dental caries and restorations are recorded. Caries, restorations, and other details are commonly recorded on a chart (Fig. 2.5). This represents the dentition when viewed from in front of the patient, so that the teeth on the right side of the page are on the patient's left and vice versa. The convention is that the horizontal line between the upper and lower teeth represents the tongue, so that the lingual or palatal surfaces are those nearest to this line, and the buccal or labial surfaces are those at the top of the top row and the bottom of the bottom row. The marks on the posterior teeth divide the tooth into occlusal, mesial, distal, buccal, and lingual surfaces, and the same applies to the anterior teeth except that there is no occlusal surface.

For reference to individual teeth, other than by using this chart, there are a number of systems of tooth notation in use. In the United Kingdom the permanent dentition is most commonly referred to by the Palmer system, in which teeth are numbered 1–8 from the midline in each quadrant. The figures when written must carry vertical and horizontal lines to indicate the quadrant: thus <u>3 2 1</u>/ to indicate the upper right (patient's right) canine, lateral incisor, and central incisor, and /4̅ to

Fig. 2.5 Conventions for charting restorations, lesions to be restored, and other conditions in the mouth.

Full description of restoration: Occlusal, Distal occlusal, Mesial occlusal, Occlusal buccal, Mesial occlusal distal, Buccal, Mesial, Mesial incisal, Buccal distal, Distal, Buccal, Palatal, Mesial occlusal buccal, Crown, Tooth missing

'Shorthand' description: O   DO   MO   OB   MOD   B   M   BD   D   B   P   MOB

Existing restorations

Right   8   7   6   5   4   3   2   1 | 1   2   3   4   5   6   7   8   Left

Treatment to be done

Lower labels: Tooth to be extracted; Occlusal restoration to be included in a new MO; MO to be included in a new MOD; To have root canal treatment; Tooth recently extracted

indicate the lower left first premolar. Deciduous teeth are given letters A–E, also from the midline.

Three other systems deserve mention. The FDI (Fédération Dentaire Internationale) system numbers the quadrants from 1 to 4 clockwise from the upper right: $\frac{1}{4}\Big|\frac{2}{3}$. This figure is added to the serial number of the tooth, so that in this notation the upper left first permanent molar is 26 (two-six) and the lower left first premolar becomes 34 (three-four). This system has the advantage that it can be easily transcribed into typescript and stored in computers, but it has the major disadvantage that it can be confused with another notation system sometimes called, quite inappropriately, the 'Universal' system which is commonly used in the United States. In this system all the teeth are given a unique number starting with the upper right third molar (1) round to the upper left third molar (16) and then clockwise round the mouth with the lower left third molar (17) and the lower right third molar (32). Thus, tooth number 16 in this system would be the upper left third molar, whereas in the FDI system it would be the upper right first molar.

To avoid this confusion and yet retain computer compatability, a system using letters and numbers is also in use. The four quadrants are designated UR (upper right), UL (upper left), LL (lower left), and LR (lower right), and the teeth are still numbered 1–8 from the midline in each quadrant. Thus, the upper right first molar would be described as UR6 and the lower left first premolar as LL4.

With the increased use of computers, the difficulty of recording the Palmer system in computers, and the significant confusion which arises between the FDI (largely European) and 'Universal' (largely United States) systems, this last system with quadrants referred to by letters has much to recommend it.

There are a number of widely used conventions for charting caries, restorations, and other changes, and some of these are shown in Fig. 2.5. Because these charts are commonly dictated to dental surgery assistants no attempt should be made to represent the size of the lesion or restoration on the chart. They are simply a shorthand notation and are not meant to be pictorially representative.

Special tests

A number of special tests may be required to supplement the information obtained from the history and examination.

Radiographs

Radiographic diagnosis of caries was dealt with in Chapter 1. Other radiographic findings relating to alveolar bone levels, periapical and other pathology, unerupted teeth, etc. should be recorded.

Vitality tests

Colour

A non-vital tooth commonly becomes darker and less translucent than the corresponding vital tooth if it is not promptly treated by removing the necrotic pulp and root filling with an inert non-staining material. If the change is slight, particularly when the tooth is heavily filled, the difference in colour may be difficult to detect. Transillumination will help to detect slight changes in colour and particularly translucency.

Presence of a sinus

A sinus over the apical region is strong evidence that there may be a necrotic pulp in a nearby tooth. Usually, but not always, the sinus discharges close to the apex of the affected tooth. If there is any doubt, and in particular when several teeth possibly have necrotic pulps, a useful investigation is to insert a gutta-percha point into the sinus (Fig. 2.6(a)) and take a radiograph (Fig. 2.6(b)). This also helps to distinguish between periapical changes arising from a necrotic pulp and pathology elsewhere, such as a lateral root canal or lateral perforation of the root by instrumentation.

Radiographs

Periapical radiographs give no direct evidence of pulp vitality. However, a periapical radiolucency usually represents a granuloma which in turn is the result of pulp necrosis. The less common periapical (radicular) cyst is also a sign of a non-vital pulp. It is not usually possible to differentiate between these two conditions from the radiographic appearance alone.

However, mistakes can be made when normal structures, such as the mental foramen, the incisal canal, or the maxillary antrum are superimposed on the root. In these cases it should be possible to trace an intact lamina dura around the normal apex. Another rare cause of periapical radiolucency, which may be associated with a tooth with a *vital* pulp, is the osteolytic phase of hypercementosis.

Thermal and electrical stimuli

The definition of pulp vitality is that the pulp retains a blood supply. Unfortunately, as yet there are no reliable means of testing the integrity of the blood supply without damaging the pulp. However, it is possible to test whether there is an intact nerve supply by thermal or electrical stimuli. Care must be taken in interpreting these second-hand results. If there is a reliable positive response to a stimulus, it can be assumed that the nerve supply is intact and therefore the blood supply must be. However, the reverse is not true; there are a number of conditions in which the nerve supply is interrupted or degenerates without losing the blood supply. This occurs after a blow, particularly in young patients, and it also occurs with extensive secondary dentine formation in teeth which have been extensively restored and in older patients.

Also, to complicate matters further, a number of patients will give false positive responses. This may be a result of anxiety about the test, fearing that it will hurt, or it

(a)

(b)

Fig. 2.6 (a) A sinus is present over the upper left central incisor and a gutta-percha point has been gently inserted into it.
(b) The radiograph of the tooth shown in (a) shows that a sinus comes from the apex of the tooth. It is possible that it might have come from a deep pocket. Extensive alveolar bone loss can be seen. The distal root caries can also be seen and this is the reason for the pulp dying.

may be that the test is badly performed so that the gingival tissues or the adjacent teeth are stimulated. In some cases it is thought that a necrotic pulp may conduct an electrical stimulus to the apical tissues, thus producing another explanation of a false positive result.

Despite these difficulties, the results of thermal and electrical stimuli are very valuable, but only when taken in conjunction with other observations.

A cold stimulus can be applied by soaking a small pledget of cotton wool in ethyl chloride which cools by rapid evaporation, and then applying this to the tooth. Alternatively, ice sticks can be made by freezing water in suitable containers. Heat can applied by warming a stick of gutta-percha, although care should be taken with this test not to damage other structures or overheat and damage a normal pulp. Occasionally a non-vital tooth may give a false positive response, possibly because the heat is conducted through the dentine to the periodontal membrane. However, a vital tooth usually responds quickly but a false positive response is slow. When carrying out electrical or thermal tests, a normal tooth is first tested to demonstrate the sensation to the patient and also to act as a basis for comparision.

Electric pulp testers (Fig. 2.7) have the advantage that initially they can be applied to the tooth with no electrical stimulus, and the current can be switched on and increased. This allows the patient to distinguish between the sensation of the tooth being touched and a stimulus applied. It also allows the test to be curtailed as soon as any sensation is felt rather than (if the pulp is already hypersensitive) suffering the application of hot or cold stimuli.

Fig. 2.7   A hand-held battery-operated pulp tester.

Percussion

Percussion tests are performed by gently tapping the crown of the tooth with a light instrument, for example the end of a mouth mirror handle. The crown should be tapped first in an axial direction and then obliquely on the buccal or lingual surfaces.

This yields *no direct evidence* of the pulpal condition. What it detects is inflammation of the periapical tissues. If these are inflamed, the tooth will act as a piston in its socket and stimulate them by pressure. The periapical tissues may be inflamed as a result of either toxins originating in a necrotic pulp or recent trauma. The tooth is described as being tender to percussion (TTP).

Instrumentation

As a last resort, a test cavity can be cut into an area of dentine that is normally sensitive. This is rarely done with an intact sound tooth, but with heavily restored, crowned, or grossly carious teeth where the vitality of the pulp is in doubt, it is common practice to start cavity preparation, or the removal of an old restoration, before giving a local anaesthetic. As soon as a sensation is felt a local anaesthetic is given; the absence of sensation increases the likelihood of the pulp being non-vital.

Finally, with all pulp testing it is important to realize that a positive response from the dental pulp does not necessarily mean that it is normal. There are no methods for detecting whether part of the pulp is damaged or necrotic, and this is particularly important in multirooted teeth.

Occlusal analysis

Sometimes a more detailed analysis of the occlusion, using articulated study casts, is useful in planning treatment. However, such analyses are expensive and time-consuming to produce, so they are not used as a routine but only when there are clear questions which are important and which can only be assessed in this way. Articulated study casts are usually required when partial dentures are designed, and, it is important that this is done at the treatment planning stage before any teeth are restored, more detailed description of functional occlusal is given by Smith (1990, Chapter 4).

Diet analysis

The past and present diet can be investigated by questioning and by completing a *diet sheet* (Fig. 1.25).

Salivary analysis

In patients with a high caries incidence, the salivary pH and buffering capacity may be tested. Also, counts of *Streptococcus mutans* and lactobacillus in the saliva may be used to monitor the caries risk and the success of a caries prevention programme (see p. 16).

THE HISTORY AND EXAMINATION PROCESS

As stressed earlier, the full history is *not* usually completed before the examination starts. Although there are many variations, a common pattern of history and examination would proceed as follows:

• reason for attendance

• medical history

• initial preliminary examination

• initial assessment of the patient's general oral and dental condition and the specific problem, if there is one

• further conversation to elicit more details of the symptoms (if there are any), and the background to the problem which is likely to be relevant—for example diet, social history, etc.

• further detailed examination

• general assessment of the patient's dental awareness and expectations

• special tests

• start the treatment planning process (see later).

Whatever sequence is used for a particular patient, it is helpful if the findings are recorded in a systematic way. The record must always be made while the patient is present, and the need for a contemporaneous record cannot be overstressed both in the interests of accuracy and also for medico-legal reasons (see later).

PLANNING THE TREATMENT

Treatment should follow a planned course in all cases. This is not to say that the plan is unalterable, and the temptation to write down a treatment plan as a prescription and then follow it without further thought or revision should be avoided. It is necessary to maintain constant vigilance for changes in the clinical circumstances, the patient's response to treatment, and the success of earlier stages in the treatment.

The general approach to treatment planning should be one of *problem solving*. This seems obvious, but is not always as simple as it sounds. One set of circumstances— for example, a mild disturbance in the appearance of a tooth—might be a real problem to one patient, causing great distress, and yet go unnoticed by another.

Cosmetic problems like this can be regarded as the *patient's* problem and he or she will ultimately decide whether they want treatment or not. Other problems are more the *dentist's*. To continue with the same example, the dentist must decide between recommending a composite restoration, a facing of composite or porcelain, or a crown. The final decision is taken jointly between patient and dentist and illustrates another important principle of treatment planning. The patient must be properly *informed* about treatment alternatives and must give *informed consent* to the treatment.

Treatment plans can conveniently be divided into 'simple' and 'complex'. A simple treatment plan is by far the most common and is all that is usually required for patients at recall visits, sometimes over many years of maintenance of a good standard of dental health. In such cases the dentist is monitoring health. However, there is a danger of both dentist and patient being lulled into a false sense of security, and it is important that at each re-examination relevant questions are asked and a proper examination made so that slow and steady development of periodontal disease or secondary caries is recognized.

A typical 'simple' treatment plan would be as follows.

1. Reinforce oral hygiene procedures lingual to lower molars.
2. Scale and polish.
3. Replace stained composites as charted (and the dental chart might show two or three anterior composites to be replaced).

A more complex treatment plan is often required for patients who have not attended for some time or where there is a need for a major reassessment of a declining state of dental health. In these cases it is helpful to divide the treatment into stages.

1. Urgent treatment for the relief of pain or other symptoms.
2. Treatment for the stabilization of progressive disease or conditions which may become acute (e.g. temporarily restore very carious teeth, remove necrotic pulps, or extract teeth even if they are symptomless at the time).
3. Assess the cause of the dental disease and begin initial preventive measures.
4. Reassess the patient's response to this initial treatment and decide the broad outline of the future plan. At this stage it may be necessary to decide between a number of alternative solutions of different complexity and cost. For example, the same clinical condition (a badly broken-down mouth with many failing restorations and unsatisfactory partial dentures) may be treated in different patients by one of the following:

   • extracting all the remaining teeth and providing complete dentures

   • providing extensive restorative treatment with multiple crowns and fixed bridges to replace the partial denture

   • a midway position between these extremes with some extractions, some restorations and new partial dentures.

   The basis of this broad decision will be the patient's motivation, his or her response to initial treatment and preventive measures, and the cost. It is a crucial decision and one of the most difficult to make. If there is any doubt, it should be deferred or, better still, a second opinion should be sought from a colleague who may be a member of the practice or the clinic or a local consultant. In some cases, for example hypodontia, decisions may need to be made about orthodontic treatment before providing veneers or crowns and bridges.

5. Provide the initial stage of definitive treatment which may be further preventive measures, periodontal treatment, orthodontic treatment, extractions, or other surgical treatment.

6. A further reassessment to evaluate the success of the first stage of treatment and revise the treatment plan as necessary.

7. Provide the final stages of the active course of treatment.

8. Reassessment, maintenance, and reinforcement of preventive measures.

The importance of making plans, both simple and complex, and of recording the decisions in the patient's record can be summarized as follows.

• It ensures that the clinician reviews the treatment in the light of all available evidence at the start of treatment and at stages throughout it.

• It is a record for later reference, particularly in complicated cases and after a lapse of time. This is available mostly for the benefit of the patient, but on occasions, when patients complain, it may have dento-legal importance and may protect the dentist against unjustified complaints. In this context, when the treatment plan is complex and expensive, it may be wise to put the advice in the form of a letter to the patient so that he or she has time to consider it and its implications before acceptance or rejection. The letter is also a written record, of which the patient has a copy, in cases where there is a dento-legal problem later.

• It avoids the risk of disorderly and ill-advised management which may arise if treatment is undertaken piecemeal. Unfortunately, this is a danger in clinics which are organized on a rigid departmental basis, so that a logical course of treatment is interupted by different lengths of waiting lists in each department or by the student's inability to carry out certain items of treatment. In a learning environment some restrictions are necessary, but it is important that the compartmentalized attitudes they engender are not carried over into practice.

SOME COMMON DECISIONS WHICH HAVE TO BE MADE

Clearly, it is not possible to to give guidance on every decision which may have to be made, but the following set of examples illustrates the nature of the decision-making process. The examples to be described are as follows:

• diagnosing toothache

• whether to restore or attempt to arrest and partially remineralize a moderately sized carious lesion and whether to restore or monitor an erosive lesion

• whether to extract or root treat a tooth

• which restorative material to use.

Other major decisions are discussed elsewhere; for example, whether caries is present or not (Chapter 1) and whether existing restorations should be replaced or not (Chapter 11).

Diagnosing toothache

This diagnosis is made almost entirely by the dentist, and although as much information as possible should be obtained, there is frequently a substantial element of judgement involved. Having made the diagnosis, again it is the dentist's job to give a prognosis, but the decision on treatment is usually shared much more equally between dentist and patient.

The patient complaining of 'toothache' is most likely to be suffering from one of the following conditions:

- acute pulpitis

- acute apical periodontitis

- acute apical abscess

- acute periodontal abscess

- exposed sensitive dentine

- food packing

- cracked cusps

- chronic pulpitis

- chronic apical periodontitis (apical granuloma).

This list of conditions is in approximate order of the severity of the pain and also of the frequency in which pain is the presenting symptom, although there are considerable individual variations in this. It is worth remembering that 'common diseases occur commonly' and that pulpitis resulting from caries is the most common cause of toothache.

There are several other painful conditions of the mouth and face which may be confused with toothache, but are not usually described by the patient as toothache, for example, maxillary sinusitis, pericoronitis, trigeminal neuralgia, mandibular dysfunction, atypical facial pain, and lesions of the salivary glands and soft tissues. However, patients with maxillary sinusitis and pericoronitis do sometimes complain of toothache, and textbooks on oral pathology and oral medicine should be consulted for descriptions òf these conditions.

The features of the nine conditions listed above are as follows.

Acute pulpitis

There is severe pain, poorly localized to the tooth, and it may not even be possible for the patient to tell whether the source of the pain is in the upper or lower jaw; however, the pain is always localized to one side or the other. To aid the clinical diagnosis and provide a basis for rational treatment planning, two clinical presentations of acute pulpitis are recognized: *reversible pulpitis* and *irreversible pulpitis*. Unfortunately, the clinical signs and symptoms of pulpitis are poorly correlated with the histological appearance of the pulp and so this is a clinical rather than a histological distinction. If the dentist considers it likely that the vitality of the pulp during treatment can be maintained the 'reversible' label will be given, whereas if he or she thinks that the pulp is damaged beyond repair the pulpitis will be considered irreversible and either root canal treatment or extraction will be the procedure of choice.

Reversible pulpitis is characterized by pain initiated by hot and cold stimuli lasting for a few seconds and disappearing when the stimulus is removed. In distinction to this, irreversible pulpitis is characterized by pain of several minutes or hours duration, also initiated and exacerbated by hot and cold stimuli but persisting long after the stimulus is removed. Alternatively, irreversible pulpitis may present as sudden *unprovoked* attacks of toothache which increase in frequency and severity but are poorly localized. In both reversible and irreversible pulpitis vitality tests may show an exaggerated response from the affected tooth, but this is not always the case. At this stage the tooth is not tender to percussion because the periapical tissues are not yet inflamed. There may be some evidence of the cause of the pulpitis, such as caries or a heavily restored tooth, but this is not a reliable way of diagnosing the affected tooth. Sometimes the tooth in the quadrant with the most obvious gross caries has been non-vital for some time and is symptomless, but another tooth with less obvious caries, perhaps under an existing restoration, is the source of the pulpitis.

Acute apical periodontitis

This is very much better localized, and the classic presenting sign is that the patient presents indicating which tooth is causing pain by gingerly pointing to it, whereas the patient with acute irreversible pulpitis holds his hand to the side of his face. The tooth will be very tender to touch, let alone percuss, and there may be some tenderness over the apex in the buccal sulcus. The pulp may retain some vitality as the periapical tissues become inflamed before the pulp finally becomes necrotic. Again, there may be caries in the crown of the tooth.

The physiological basis for this accurate localization of the pain by the patient compared with poor localization with pulpitis is that the pulp contains *pain* nerve endings only, but the periodontal ligament contains both *pain and pressure-sensitive* nerve endings. Therefore in acute pulpitis, only poorly localized pain is felt, whereas in acute apical periodontitis pain is felt *and* movement of the tooth stimulates the pressure-sensitive nerve endings and identifies the affected tooth.

Acute apical abscess

The patient will usually present with a large tender swelling, either intra-orally or on the face, although sometimes the patient presents before the swelling has appeared or after it has spontaneously burst or subsided. The spread of infection from the apices of teeth follows well-defined patterns which are described in textbooks of oral surgery. For example, an acute apical abcess on an upper lateral incisor commonly points onto the palate, whereas on the upper canine tooth it points facially and causes swelling of the cheek and may close the eye. The tooth will be very tender to touch and the patient will often not be prepared to close his teeth together. The patient may also feel unwell and have a temperature. By this stage the pulp will usually give a non-vital response, although pulp tests are unreliable in view of the patient's distress.

Acute periodontal abscess

An acute periodontal (or lateral) abscess forms at the base of a deep periodontal pocket. The presentation is similar to that for acute apical periodontitis or acute apical abscess but the tooth may still be vital. This is because the inflammation is not the consequence of spread of infection from a necrotic pulp.

Exposed sensitive dentine

This may result from gingival recession or surgery producing exposed root surfaces, or it may result from a failing restoration or caries exposing dentine to oral fluids. The patient will usually complain of sensitivity to hot, cold, and *sweet* food and drink, but the sensitivity (rather than pain) is often poorly localized. It may indeed be generalized in several areas of the mouth. Pulp tests applied to enamel surfaces will produce a normal response, but if the exposed dentine surface is stimulated either thermally or electrically, or is scratched with a probe, there may be an increased response. The teeth are not tender to percussion.

Food packing

When the contact point between adjacent teeth is not tight, either as a result of the teeth drifting apart or because of a poorly contoured restoration, food wedges between the teeth and causes periodontal pain. Meat fibres are the most troublesome.

Cracked cusps

Cusps may crack either superficially or deep into the tooth, whether the tooth is restored or not. The crack may involve the pulp or pass only through enamel and dentine. The symptoms are often poorly localized and may occur only periodically. Sometimes there is a sharp pain on biting hard on tough food, and occasionally with thermal stimuli. Thermal and electrical pulp tests are often inconclusive and the tooth may not be tender to percussion although pressure laterally on individual cusps may produce pain. Transillumination may help to show the crack, or applying disclosing solution or other stain to the tooth may reveal it. Unfortunately, many teeth show multiple cracks and do not cause symptoms (perhaps because these cracks only involve enamel), and thus it is difficult to be sure that any crack that is seen is actually the cause of the pain (Fig. 2.8). A useful diagnostic test is to ask the patient to bite on a cotton-wool roll. Pain is often felt when the pressure is *released* rather than when it is *applied*. Sometimes, when the restoration is removed from a suspect tooth, the crack is seen at the base of the cavity and these deep cracks are more likely to cause symptoms (Fig. 2.9).

Fig. 2.8 Cracks are obvious in the distal and lingual walls. Lateral pressure on the disto-lingual cusp caused pain but pressure on the other cusps did not. (Reproduced by courtesy of Mr D. W. Bartlett.)

Chronic pulpitis

This produces mild poorly localized pain which sometimes comes and goes over a period of weeks or months. Eventually, if untreated, the pulp usually dies and the symptoms of chronic pulpitis disappear, although symptoms of periapical changes may take over. The tooth will usually respond to vitality tests and will not be tender to percussion. With poor localization and the absence of positive signs, this is one of the most difficult conditions to diagnose. However, it is often possible to reach the general conclusion that chronic pulpitis is the most likely cause of the symptoms. If the pain is not too severe, no treatment should be given initially other than reviewing the patient frequently and waiting for the chronic pulpitis to recover, which it may well do if it is the result of caries which has been treated. Alternatively the pulp may die, in which case regular vitality tests may localize the condition to one tooth and the pulp remnants can be removed. If the pain is more severe, the causative tooth can be found only by removing restorations from the teeth one at a time and dressing the teeth with sedative materials until the symptoms disappear (see Chapter 3). Sometimes, on removing the restorations, previously unrecognized caries or a cracked cusp is revealed and this is the cause of the chronic pulpitis.

Fig. 2.9. A cracked tooth. The restoration was removed and the base of the cavity stained with disclosing solution before the tooth was extracted. The disclosing solution demonstrated the presence of this deep crack which inevitably involves the pulp. (Reproduced by courtesy of Professor A. H. R. Rowe.)

Chronic apical periodontitis

This is usually a symptomless condition, although the patient may feel a very mild pain on biting. Vitality tests will be negative, and the tooth may be slightly tender to vigorous percussion and may emit a slightly duller sound. The patient may present with a sinus. However, the main diagnostic test is a periapical radiograph on which a periapical radiolucency is seen. When a sinus is present a gutta-percha point may be gently inserted into it before the radiograph is taken and the resulting film will show this point approaching the apex of the relevant tooth. In all the other conditions listed so far, there is no radiographic change in the periapical tissues except a slight thickening of the apical periodontal space with an acute apical abscess owing to the intense pressure in the area which extrudes the tooth slightly from its socket.

In its chronic state, an apical granuloma is not infected with bacterial organisms but is a chronic inflammatory response to toxins leaching from the apex of a tooth with a necrotic pulp. These toxins percolate through the granulation tissue and become diluted and absorbed, so that there is a natural limit to the size of a chronic periapical granuloma. Beyond this size the toxins become too dilute to stimulate the formation of osteoclasts and the removal of bone.

A periapical granuloma is highly vascular because granulation tissue is essentially a repair tissue. If the necrotic pulp is removed and the tooth root filled, the granuloma will be replaced by normal bone (Fig. 2.10).

(a)

(b)

(c)

Two changes can occur within a chronic apical granuloma: it may become infected and flare up into an acute apical abscess, or it may become cystic. The clinical signs of acute change are those of an acute apical abscess, although the radiograph will show a periapical radiolucency. Similarly, the cyst may become infected and flare up into an acute apical abscess. These changes are described in textbooks of oral pathology, and the management is described in textbooks of endodontics and oral surgery.

Fig. 2.10 (a) The pulp of the second premolar tooth has become necrotic and a periapical granuloma has formed.
(b) Immediately after root filling.
(c) Three years later periapical bone has reformed. (Reproduced by courtesy of Dr. T. R. Pitt Ford.)

Making the diagnosis

Although it is necessary to know the characteristic symptoms and signs of each of the conditions listed above, it is also necessary to have a systematic method of diagnosing the cause of symptoms in a patient with toothache.

The history should concentrate on the nature of the pain, its duration, and initiating stimuli. Clues should be followed; for example, chronic sensitivity to sweet foods may suggest exposed dentine rather than any of the other conditions, and chronic tenderness to biting will suggest either a cracked cusp or perhaps chronic apical periodontitis. The past dental history may be of interest in cases where trauma or recent restorations may be the cause.

On examining the patient, the dentist should look for possible causes such as caries, leaking restorations, cracked cusps, or evidence of trauma. Radiographs, vitality tests, and percussion tests are all required in order to be confident of a diagnosis in almost every case. Radiographs may show periapical radiolucencies, failed root fillings, internal or external root resorption, fractured roots, and other possible reasons for the toothache. The value of vitality and percussion tests is clear from the earlier descriptions.

Figure 2.11 shows the typical interpretation of signs and symptoms in toothache.

Finally, despite having completed a full investigation, there are occasions when the cause of the pain is still not clear. At this point it is wise to reconsider other causes of pain, such as trigeminal neuralgia, but if these can safely be eliminated then, and only then, the dentist should start to remove previous restorations.

	Acute Pulpitis	Acute apical periodontitis	Acute apical abscess	Acute periodontal abscess	Exposed sensitive dentine	Food packing	Cracked cusp	Chronic Pulpitis	Chronic apical periodontitis (Apical granuloma)
History	Recent pain with hot and cold. May be very severe. Poorly localized.	Tender to bite. Well localized.	Pain and swelling. Very well localized.	Localized swelling. Some pain.	Generalised pain to hot, cold and sweet.	Pain after eating fibrous food, e.g. meat.	Vague intermittent pain usually on biting. May be poorly localized.	Vague, unprovoked intermittent but increasing pain. Poorly localized.	May have had pain in the past. Now not sensitive to hot and cold.
Clinical examination	Possibly caries or recent large restoration.	Possibly caries.	May be extra-oral or intra-oral swelling over apex of tooth.	Intra-oral swelling nearer to gingival margin. Tooth may be mobile.	Gingival recession. Exposed dentine at the gingival margin. Sensitive to probe or cold air.	Open contact points. Gingival inflammation. Food usually present.	Often nothing, but crack may be seen. May be painful with occlusal contact only.	May have large restoration or caries.	May have large restoration or caries.
Vitality test	Hypersensitive.	May still be vital, but usually non-vital.	Non-vital.	Often vital.	Vital.	May be vital or non-vital.	May be hypersensitive.	Often normal but may be hypersensitive.	Non-vital.
Percussion	Not tender.	Tender.	Tender to touch. Too tender to percuss.	Slight tenderness, more to lateral than axial pressure.	Not tender.	Not tender to percussion. May be sore with lateral percussion.	Usually not tender but may be.	Not tender.	Slightly. May give dull sound on percussion.
Other clinical tests			Raised temperature. Looks ill.	Deep pockets. Pus may be released on probing pocket.		Floss passes the contact easily.	Sometimes tender to lateral pressure on an individual cusp.		
Radiographic findings	Probably caries close to pulp. No periapical change.	Usually no periapical change in the early stage.	Usually no periapical change except slight thickening of apical periodontal membrane.	Alveolar bone loss. Usually no periapical change.	May be some alveolar bone loss.	None.	None.	None.	Periapical radiolucency.
Findings on further investigations	Carious exposure of pulp.	Necrotic pulp.	Pus may be drained via access cavity to root canal without local anaesthetic giving immediate relief of pain and confirming the diagnosis.				Crack sometimes visible at base of cavity when old restoration removed. If left, cuspal fracture will eventually occur.	Symptoms may settle if restoration removed and tooth dressed with calcium hydroxide, but pulp often dies eventually.	Necrotic pulp.

Fig. 2.11 Typical signs and symptoms in toothache. Unfortunately, not all symptoms fall precisely into this pattern and clinical judgement and experience is often needed for their interpretation.

A simplistic maxim, but one well worth remembering, is 'diagnosis should precede treatment'. Far too often busy dentists, pressed for time, feel an obligation to start treating teeth without having made a thorough diagnosis of the cause of the toothache.

Whether to restore or attempt to arrest and partially remineralize a moderate-size carious lesion and whether to restore or monitor an erosive lesion

With caries this decision will primarily be the dentist's, but with an erosive lesion the patient will often be much more involved in the decision.

Guidance is given in Chapter 1 as to when, in general, caries should be removed and the tooth restored, and when measures should be taken to partially remineralize the tooth. These general guidelines must now be applied to the individual patient. The factors to be considered will include the age and previous caries experience of the patient. The social history may also be important in that if the patient is able (and likely) to come for regular examinations then it is better to give even reasonably advanced lesions the chance to arrest and partially remineralize, whereas with a patient who is going away for a year or two the opposite decision is likely to be made.

With a carious lesion the main problem in making this decision is to decide the prognosis. This is also the problem in deciding what to do about an erosive lesion, but in this case the consequences of not treating the lesion are likely to be less rapid if the wrong decision is made. It is possible to see the full extent of the erosive lesion, and pulp exposure arising from dental erosion is very uncommon. With caries the extent of the lesion within the tooth is less clear, and if the wrong decision is made and the caries develops rapidly then pulpitis may ensue. This is part of the reason why the patient can be more involved in the decision as to whether to restore an erosive lesion. The primary reasons for restoring these lesions are as follows.

- They spoil the patient's appearance (this is the patient's decision not the dentist's).

- They are sensitive in a way that cannot be controlled by topical agents (again, only the patient knows how sensitive they are and how much he or she can tolerate).

- The dentist may be concerned about the weakening or other mechanical effects of allowing the lesion to progress.

Whether to extract or root treat a tooth

Again, the patient is often very much involved with this decision. Some patients (a rapidly declining number) will opt to have a painful or broken-down tooth extracted on the grounds of time involved in treatment, fear of treatment, lack of confidence that root treatment is likely to be successful, or cost. This is particularly likely with a tooth which does not show and which may appear to the patient not to have any great value. In this case, if the tooth is painful or grossly carious or has a necrotic pulp, the dentist should comply with the patient's wish for an extraction even though he/she may feel sure that the tooth can be saved with a good prognosis and that this is the treatment he/she would strongly advise. It would not be ethical to leave the patient in pain when a simple form of treatment, such as extraction, would reliably relieve it and the patient will not accept other forms of treatment.

However, most patients are willing to accept the dentist's advice. Advice should be based on the general long-term interest of the patient rather than on an oversimplified wish to retain all teeth at all costs. For example, pulpitis in a first molar tooth in a child with crowded arches may well be best treated by extraction followed by balancing extractions or by orthodontic treatment to close the space and relieve the crowding, even if this is not the ideal tooth to extract for orthodontic purposes. In contrast, posterior teeth, notably second and third molars, are particularly valuable if a partial denture may have to be worn. This is because a denture is much more stable if it has a posterior abutment tooth to retain and support it.

Finally, it must be remembered that some teeth cannot be saved because of gross caries, and even though root canal treatment may be possible, it is not advisable because it will not be possible to restore a healthy functional crown.

Which restorative material to use

Much of the answer to this will become apparent in later chapters. However, decisions made now with the current state of development of restorative materials will alter, probably quite rapidly in the next few years. This has certainly been the case to a very considerable extent since the first edition of this book, and so it is important that the decisions made in a given set of circumstances do not become fossilized in the dentist's mind so that he or she continues to use the same materials and the same techniques long after they have been replaced by improved materials and techniques. There is a happy medium between seizing on every new material which comes on to the market and assuming that it will outperform all its predecesors, and retaining too conservative a view, being unprepared to use new materials until they have survived long-term clinical trials.

FURTHER READING

Besford, J. (1986). *Good mouth keeping*. Oxford University Press.

Elderton, R. J. (ed.) (1987). *Positive dental prevention*. Heinemann, London.

Scully, C. and Cawson, R. A. (1993). *Medical problems in dentistry* (3rd edn). John Wright, Bristol.

Smith, B. G. N. (1990). Planning and making crowns and bridges, Chapter 4. Martin Dunitz, London.

3 Principles of cavity design and preparation

G. V. BLACK

In the first decade of this century an American dentist and teacher, G. V. Black, established principles governing the design of cavities and suggested steps in their preparation. He based these principles on what was known at the time about the natural history of caries and the restorative materials available. The wisdom of his work was such that it remained virtually unchallenged for more than half a century. Now, with new materials, a better understanding of caries, and research findings into the success or otherwise of various restorative procedures, the principles have been largely revised.

G. V. Black was a far-sighted scientist who would surely have expected that his ideas would have been taken up, researched, and revised by successive generations of clinicians and scientists. It would perhaps have been a disappointment to him that this was not done until relatively recently, but he would undoubtedly have been the first to applaud these developments. In 1908 Dr Black wrote 'the complete divorcement of dental practice from studies of the pathology of dental caries, that existed in the past, is an anomaly in science that should not continue. It has the apparent tendency plainly to make dentists mechanics only.'

Since his principles have now been so extensively modified, and since many conditions in addition to caries are treated operatively (see Chapter 1), no further reference will be made to Black's principles.

Black also described a classification of carious lesions which is still widely used in dental schools. However, this classification is now regarded as incomplete in that it does not include root caries and secondary caries. Also, it does not include non-carious lesions, which are treated in the same way as carious lesions. Therefore this classification is not used in this book but it is a useful clinical shorthand and is as follows:

- Class I. Caries affecting pits and fissures.
- Class II. Caries affecting the approximal surfaces of posterior teeth.
- Class III. Caries affecting the approximal surfaces of anterior teeth.
- Class IV. Caries affecting the approximal surfaces of anterior teeth and involving the incisal angle.
- Class V. Caries affecting the cervical surfaces.

WHY RESTORE TEETH?

The objectives of restoring teeth are as follows:
- to remove diseased tissue as necessary
- to restore the integrity of the tooth surface
- to restore the function of the tooth
- to restore the appearance of the tooth.

WHAT DETERMINES CAVITY DESIGN?

The general principles of cavity design are related to the following:

- the structure and properties of the dental tissues
- the diseases (e.g. caries, pathological tooth wear, periodontal disease)
- the properties of the restorative materials.

The dental tissues

Enamel, the hardest tissue in the body, is relatively inelastic and rather brittle. Its structure consists of interlinked rods and it is thought to have a greater tendency to split along the line of the rods than in other directions. For this reason unsupported enamel to which occlusal forces are applied directly should usually be removed so that it does not fracture and leave a gap between the restoration and the tooth. However, elsewhere unsupported enamel may be left, particularly when the restoration is to be in a composite or glass ionomer material since these materials bond to the dental tissues and thus give them some support. The risk to unsupported enamel where there are no direct occlusal forces is from the restorative procedure itself; for example, tightening a matrix band (see p. 123) may damage unsupported enamel at a cervical margin.

Dentine is softer, more porous, and more elastic than enamel and is sensitive. The elasticity of dentine allows the use of pins, which may help to retain a restoration and which can be screwed into a slightly undersized hole. If this were attempted in enamel it would split; imagine putting a wood screw into a pre-drilled hole in wood compared with glass.

In a vital tooth dentine is intimately connected with the pulp, being permeated by tubules which contain the cytoplasmic extensions of the odontoblasts at their pulpal ends. For this reason dentine and pulp are often considered together. This intimate connection between the two tissues means that diseases or operative procedures that affect the dentine may also affect the pulp.

The shape, size, and condition of the pulp will affect cavity design. In a slowly progressing carious lesion, reparative dentine within the pulp chamber will have reduced the size of the pulp so that in some cases the cavity will extend into the contours of the original pulp chamber (Fig. 3.1). However, in most cases the preparation is designed to avoid the pulp. In all cases, precautions are taken to avoid physical, thermal, or chemical damage to the pulp during cavity preparation and placing the restoration.

The gingival tissues become inflamed in the presence of plaque, and so cavities are designed and restorations placed in such a way that minimal encroachment upon the gingival attachment occurs, and also so that the margins of restorations are as easy to clean as possible. This also helps to reduce the likelihood of secondary caries.

Fig. 3.1 A hemisection of an extracted tooth to show reparative dentine reducing the size of the pulp chamber. However, the caries has now progressed into this reparative dentine.

The diseases

The effect of caries, tooth wear, trauma, and defects in tooth structure have been described in Chapter 1. The implications of these must be considered in designing cavities. For example, the spread of caries along the enamel-dentine junction undermines the enamel and has an important influence over cavity design. Near the pulp the distinction between infected carious dentine and dentine which has been affected by caries, but which does not yet contain bacteria, is important in deciding how much to remove. Of particular importance is the fact that restorations can only repair the cavities cut to remove carious lesions, and preventive measures such as dietary advice, judicious use of fluoride, and good plaque control are essential if restorations are to last.

Similarly, in cases of extensive tooth wear the proportions of erosion, attrition, and abrasion contributing to the tooth wear must be diagnosed, if possible, and the success of preventive measures assessed before the teeth are restored. If further tooth wear cannot be prevented, the rate at which the condition is likely to progress will affect the choice of restoration and its design. For example, if the main cause of tooth wear is acid regurgitation which cannot be prevented medically or surgically, the dentist may need to consider crowning the teeth so that they last as long as possible in these adverse circumstances.

The properties of the restorative materials

The materials currently used to restore teeth which will be described in this book are as follows:

- dental amalgam

- composite resins

- glass ionomer cements

- cast gold and other alloys

- porcelain.

Other materials such as silicate cement, acrylic resin, and cohesive gold are no longer used to any extent and materials used for crowns and bridges are not described in this book.

When considering dental materials it is useful to have some concept of an ideal material. Unfortunately, this dental paragon does not exist, but scientists are continually striving to improve dental materials and enormous strides have been made since the first edition of this book.

The ideal material would have the following properties:

- be easy to use

- be tooth-coloured

- be adhesive to tooth substance

- have no change of volume on setting

- provide protection from recurrent caries

- have adequate strength

- be insoluble and non-corrodible in the mouth

- be non-toxic and non-irritant to pulp and gingival tissues

- be easy to trim and polish

- resist the formation of dental plaque

- have a rate of wear similar to enamel

- have a coefficient of thermal expansion similar to enamel and dentine

- have a thermal diffusivity similar to enamel and dentine

- have a low water absorption

- be radiopaque

- have a good shelf life

- be inexpensive.

While the relevance of some of these ideal properties is obvious, others need a word of explanation. Adhesion to tooth substance is desirable, so that the filling may give some support to the tooth and be retained within it. In addition, any adhesive material should minimize the gap between restoration and tooth that would invite secondary caries (see p. 9) and may make it unecessary to produce retentive features in a cavity. A volume change in a material as it sets is a problem because expansion may fracture the tooth and contraction may open up a gap between the filling and the cavity wall. Since recurrent caries may occur around restorations, a material which exerts some cariostatic or bactericidal effect is useful.

The mouth is a highly hostile environment for any material, being warm, wet, and full of bacteria which potentially may cause disease. In addition, the temperature of the mouth is not constant, since hot and cold food and drinks transiently pass through it. This means that the cavity seal of a material may be lost unless it has a thermal diffusivity and coefficient of thermal expansion that are similar to enamel and dentine.

The ideal material would resist plaque formation and would be capable of accurate finishing to a smooth lustrous surface which is easily cleaned and which would not dissolve, corrode, or wear excessively in service. Radiopacity is important in the diagnosis of recurrent caries on radiographs (see p. 184).

A textbook of dental materials should be consulted to study the composition, setting reactions, and properties of the materials described in this book. Advances in materials science have had a profound effect on operative techniques, making the study of dental materials particularly relevant and important to today's graduate. The following brief description of some of the relevant clinical properties of materials is given to illustrate the effect they have on cavity preparation.

Dental amalgam

Amalgam is an alloy of mercury with silver and other metals such as tin and copper to give a set material which does not adhere to tooth structure and therefore needs to be retained within the cavity by mechanical means. It has adequate strength in bulk but is brittle in small sections and so it is necessary to design cavities so that amalgam margins are in excess of 70 degrees (Figs 3.2(a) and 3.2(b)) (see Chapter 6).

It is not tooth-coloured and therefore is used only in posterior teeth where its strength, abrasion resistance, and ability to retain a good polish still make it a popular material.

Although amalgam does not adhere to the tooth surface, it has been shown that there is a reduction in microleakage around amalgam restorations over a period of time, and this is attributed to corrosion products forming at the tooth-amalgam interface.

Amalgam is condensed into a cavity with more force than other materials and this must be resisted by the design of the cavity preparation.

Composition of amalgam alloys and its relevance to clinical practice
When the alloy was originally formulated the major components were silver (65 per cent), tin (29 per cent), and copper (6 per cent). Thus a silver–tin intermetallic compound (Ag_3Sn), known as the gamma (γ) phase, predominated strengthened by a small amount of copper. However, modern amalgam alloys now contain more copper (10–30 per cent instead of 6 per cent). These *copper-enriched* alloys also contain small quantities of other metals such as palladium. The high copper alloys have two important advantages over the original formulation and both affect the marginal adaptation of the set material. Set amalgams undergo a certain amount of plastic deformation or *creep* when subjected to stress such as occlusal stress. Creep causes the set amalgam to flow over the margins of the cavity to give an unsupported edge, which may be further weakened by *corrosion* of the alloy. Fracture of this edge

Enamel

Dentine

Amalgam

(a)

Amalgam
or
composite

(b)

Composite

(c)

Composite

(d)

Fig. 3.2 (a) An amalgam restoration prepared and carved so that the amalgam margin angle is too acute. This increases the likelihood of fracture of the amalgam margin.
(b) The amalgam margin angle has been increased by altering both the preparation and carving. The same margin can be used for composite restorations.
(c) The enamel margin is sometimes bevelled when composite is used.
(d) Alternatively, when dentine caries undermines the enamel, the enamel may be left undercut provided that it is not subjected to direct occlusal forces.

may form a *ditch* around the margin of the filling (see p. 180). Copper-enriched alloys exhibit less creep and less corrosion than the original alloys, and clinical trials show that they are less prone to ditching. Since an objective of operative dentistry is to produce a smooth and therefore easily cleaned junction between the filling and the tooth, this is an important advantage and explains why the earlier alloys have been replaced by the copper-enriched type.

Sometimes a small amount of zinc is used as a scavenger during the production of an alloy. If a zinc-containing alloy is contaminated with moisture during condensation, the zinc reacts with water producing hydrogen. This causes a delayed expansion of the alloy which may produce pain. For this reason moisture control is important when placing these materials.

The shape and size of alloy particles varies from one product to another because two different methods are used to manufacture the particles. They may be cut from a prehomogenized ingot of alloy; this produces *lathe-cut* alloy powders with particles of irregular shape that are then graded according to size. Alternatively, the particles may be produced by atomization, where the molten alloy is sprayed into a column filled with inert gas. The droplets of alloy solidify in a *spherical* form as they fall down the column. The shape of the alloy particles (lathe-cut or spherical) is relevant to the dentist using the material. Spherical alloys require less force (condensation pressure) to push them into position. Some alloys use a combination of shapes and sizes of particle.

High copper levels in alloy powders are produced by the manufacturer in a number of ways. The ratio of metals may be adjusted at the melting stage and either lathe-cut or spherical powders produced. These are called *single-composition copper-enriched alloys*. Another approach is to blend particles of a conventional alloy with those of a silver-copper alloy to achieve a higher overall copper content. These blends are called *dispersion-modified copper-enriched alloys*. One widely used product contains two parts by weight of a lathe-cut alloy containing less than 6 per cent copper and one part by weight of spherical silver–copper eutectic particles (28 per cent copper). The final copper content in the blended alloy is 12 per cent. Since the alloy is a mixture of lathe-cut and spherical particles it will handle more like the former than the latter, requiring considerable packing pressure for condensation.

It can be seen that practitioners have a number of alloys to choose from but should always know which alloy they are using. The choice of alloy will have a bearing on both the clinical handling and the long-term performance of the restorative material.

The safety of amalgam

The controversy over the safety of amalgam restorations is an important subject that is currently receiving much attention in the news media. The topic is raised at regular intervals, and all dentists should be conversant with the latest scientific literature so that the matter can be discussed with patients in an informed manner. Details of a review article by Eley and Cox (1993) are given at the end of the chapter.

There is concern over the safety of amalgam because of the mercury it contains which could be released when a filling is placed, during the functional life of a restoration, or during its removal. Scientific groups throughout the world have investigated the safety of amalgam, and there is no evidence that the *minute amount* of mercury released from dental amalgams contributes to systemic disease or has any systemic toxological effects. There is no justification for discontinuing the use of dental amalgam as a filling material or recommending replacement of existing amalgam fillings. Specifically, there is no proven relationship between amalgam and multiple sclerosis, Alzheimer's disease, myalgic encephalitis, or migraine.

There has also been concern about the possible effects of mercury from amalgam restorations in pregnancy. Human studies show no correlation between the surface area of amalgam restorations and mercury levels in maternal blood, amniotic fluid, milk, or neonatal blood.

However, there is no doubt that *high* levels of mercury are toxic and dental practitioners must handle it with care so that the local and general environment is not contaminated with either mercury or waste amalgam. Entrapment filters should be fitted to drainage systems to prevent amalgam waste reaching the sewage system, and waste amalgam should be collected and kept under reducing agents such as photographic fixer. Strict mercury and amalgam hygiene procedures should be observed in amalgam preparation, placement, removal, and polishing to minimize the mercury exposure of staff and patients.

Nevertheless it is important to put the role of dental amalgam in environmental mercury pollution into context. A report in 1992 by the United States Environmental Protection Agency showed that in 1989 discarded household batteries accounted for 86 per cent of waste mercury while dental amalgam represented only 0.56 per cent. This amount is tiny when compared with other sources of pollution and has actually decreased by 75 per cent in the last 20 years, demonstrating the awareness and response of the profession to the possible hazard.

The preceding paragraphs all deal with the *toxicity* of mercury. Everybody— patients, ancillary staff, and dentists—is susceptible to the toxic effects of mercury. In addition, a very small number of people are genuinely *allergic* to mercury. The number of reported cases which have been confirmed by properly controlled allergy testing is only a few dozen worldwide. However, some patients consider that a very wide range of symptoms of which they complain should be attributed to mercury allergy. In many cases no allergy is confirmed when these patients are tested. However, the possibility must be taken seriously, and if the patient is sufficiently concerned and the symptoms are such that it is conceivable that they may be due to mercury allergy, he or she should be referred for proper allergy testing.

Following each round of media attention to this subject many dentists are asked by patients to remove all their amalgam fillings and replace them with alternative materials. These requests should usually be kindly and gently resisted with a full explanation of the difference between toxicity and allergy which many patients find difficult to understand.

Composite resins

There are several groups of composite resin materials; although most are tooth-coloured, some have been designed for use in anterior teeth, where appearance is most important, while others have been designed for posterior teeth where strength and abrasion resistance are of prime importance. In both cases the material is capable of being attached physically to the enamel by means of the acid-etch technique. Composite is strong in thin section when attached to enamel and so the enamel margins can be bevelled, prepared with a cavo-surface angle of 90 degrees or undercut (Figs 3.2(b), 3.2(c) and 3.2(d)).

Composite resins can be attached to dentine by chemical bonding materials or via an intermediate layer of glass ionomer cement. Unfortunately, the bond to dentine is not as strong as the bond to enamel. Since the material shrinks as it sets, there is a danger that it will move away from the dentine towards the enamel in cavities bounded by enamel on one side and dentine on the other, as commonly occurs with cervical cavities. This invites recurrent caries on the dentine side of the cavity. This problem is reduced by packing the material into the cavity in special ways (see Chapters 6–9).

Composition of composite resins

All composites are a mixture of a resin and a filler. The two commonly used *resins* are either BIS GMA or urethane dimethacrylate. BIS GMA resin is made by a reaction between bisphenol A and glycidylmethacrylate, but this resin has the consistency of thick treacle at room temperature. Therefore the manufacturers use a diluent monomer (triethylene glycol dimethacrylate (TEGMA) to reduce the viscosity and allow the filler particles to be added to the resin.

The type, concentration, particle size, and particle-size distribution of the *filler* used in a commercial composite material are major factors controlling the properties and handling characteristics of the material. Fillers include quartz, fused silicon, and various types of glass including aluminosilicates and borosilicates. Some contain barium oxide to make the material radiopaque. Radiopaque materials must always be chosen for posterior teeth so that the material can be distinguished from dental caries on radiographs.

Conventional composites contain 60–80 per cent by weight of quartz or glass particles of sizes ranging from 1 to 50 μm. Manufacturers coat the filler particles with a silane *coupling agent* to enhance bonding between the filler and the resin matrix.

Particle-size distribution may vary within the range given above from one composite to another. The more modern materials contain larger quantities of smaller particles (1–5 μm), making the material easier to smooth and polish.

The search for a polishable material led to the introduction of a group of materials called *micro-filled composites* which contained silica particles with a mean diameter of only 0.04 μm. Initially it proved impossible to incorporate high filler loadings in these materials and this led to inadequate physical properties. The manufacturers solved this problem by making prepolymerized blocks of resin containing a high filler loading of silica. These blocks were ground up to give particles of resin-silica which were then mixed into more resin to form pastes of appropriate viscosity for clinical use.

A third series of composite materials contain a blend of both conventional glass or quartz particles together with some submicron particulate silica. These products are referred to as *hybrid* composites and a total filler content of 80–90 per cent by weight can be achieved.

Polymerization of composite resins

Polymerization can be activated *chemically* by mixing two components (usually two pastes), one of which contains an initiator and the other an activator. Alternatively, polymerization can be activated by exposure to *visible light*. These light-cured materials are supplied as a single paste and require the use of a specialist light source. Care must be taken to protect the dispensed material by a light-proof cover, since exposure to sunlight, or the surgery operating light, may initiate polymerization, causing the paste to thicken and become unworkable. Light-cured materials give the clinician a longer working time but great care must be taken to build the material up in increments that are not too thick. If too thick an increment is placed, the material at the base of the cavity will not set because the light cannot reach it. This leaves the clinician in a fool's paradise thinking that a restoration is satisfactory because it has a hard surface concealing a 'soggy bottom'!

Glass ionomer cements

Glass ionomer cement is the most recently developed restorative material in general use. It adheres chemically to enamel and dentine. Since it links to calcium ions in the dental tissues, the bond to enamel is stronger than the bond to dentine because enamel is more highly mineralized. However, the chemical bond of glass ionomer to enamel is not as strong as the physical bond of composite to acid-etched enamel.

Traditional, autocuring, glass ionomer cements

Glass ionomer cements (or glass polyalkenoate cements) are *water based*. They consist of an *aluminosilicate glass* with a high fluoride content which reacts with a *poly(alkenoic acid)*. The resulting cement consists of glass particles surrounded and supported by a matrix arising from the dissolution of the surface of the glass particles in the acid. *Calcium* polyacrylate chains form quite rapidly when the cement is mixed and this develops a matrix that holds the particles together. Now *aluminium* ions begin to form aluminium polyacrylate chains which are less soluble and stronger, and the final matrix formation takes place. *Fluoride*, which is used as a flux in the manufacture of the glass particles, is released from those particles and lies free within the matrix but plays no part in its physical make-up. Thus, the fluoride is able to leach out of the restoration and return to it, so that the restoration can be regarded as a *fluoride reservoir*.

Approximately 24 per cent of the set cement is water, some of which is 'loosely bound' and easily removed by dehydration. The rest is 'tightly bound' water which cannot be removed and remains an important part of the setting reaction. In the early stages after mixing the calcium polyacrylate chains remain highly soluble in water so that further water can be taken up. Conversely, the loosely bound water can be lost by evaporation if the cement is exposed to air. This problem of initial water loss or water uptake is critical to the cement and explains why it is essential to protect the surface of the newly set material with a layer of resin. A careful matrix technique should be used because finishing techniques, other than minimal carving with sharp instruments, must be delayed to a subsequent appointment by which time the material will have fully matured.

Glass ionomer cements are routinely used with conditioning agents (a 10 second application of 10 per cent polyacrylic acid) to remove part of the smear layer. This is important to achieve the optimum adhesive bond.

The properties of glass ionomer cements—adhesion to tooth structure, fluoride release, and fluoride uptake—make them ideal restorative materials for the restoration of non-load-bearing surfaces and erosion lesions, and as materials of choice for the stabilization of carious lesions. However, they are not strong enough to resist occlusal forces.

'Cermet' is a version of glass ionomer cement which contains silver powder. This is claimed to give the material greater abrasion resistance, although it is still not sufficiently strong to replace the approximal marginal ridge on a posterior tooth. Since the silver particles destroy the tooth-like appearance of the material, it is only used in posterior teeth. However, the silver gives it a radiopacity which is an advantage, because it is impossible to detect secondary caries radiographically adjacent to radiolucent materials.

Resin-modified glass ionomer cement
A new generation of glass ionomer cements which form a continuum between traditional autocured glass ionomer cements and composite resins is now available. It is important to realize that not all these materials are the same. Some are still glass ionomer cements containing resins. These materials show the fluoride release and fluoride uptake of a traditional glass ionomer cement. The set of the resin component is light initiated, but the set and maturation of the glass ionomer components continue after light exposure. These materials will set in the dark and do not give unlimited working time. It is not strictly correct to describe them as light-cured glass ionomer cements; *resin-modified glass ionomer cements* is a more accurate term.

The resin addition makes these materials apparently more user-friendly than the traditional glass ionomer cements. Initial water balance is not so critical and finishing can be done at once, rather than delaying to a subsequent appointment. The resin in the material will bind chemically to composite resin which would appear to make these materials ideal for some of the layered glass ionomer–composite restorations described later in this text.

However, the materials are still very new and have yet to be evaluated fully. All light-cured materials shrink on setting, but the shrinkage stresses in these materials are relieved by water uptake. It is possible that the resin in the new materials may cause hydrolytic instability and colour change over time.

Compomers
Compomers are also materials which contain glass ionomer components, but they are principally composite resins. These materials do not set in the dark, and this simple test will enable a practitioner to differentiate a resin-modified glass ionomer material from one which is principally a composite resin. At the time of writing the manufacturers call these materials *compomers*, and there is currently discussion as to whether they will release sufficient fluoride to simulate the cariostatic properties of the traditional glass ionomer cements.

Cast gold and other alloys
The advantage of cast metal is that it is strong in thin sections and can be used to protect weakened tooth structure. This property is the major reason for using cast metal restorations, and so cavities are designed so that weakened cusps are protected by a layer of metal. The cavity is prepared in such a way that the restoration (an inlay) is made outside the mouth and then cemented into the cavity.

At one time the small gold inlay was a popular restoration and innumerable inlays have served well for many decades. However, they cannot now be regarded as cost-effective by comparison with improved amalgam and other restorative materials and so are seldom made by most dentists. In the United Kingdom National Health Service less than one in a thousand restorations is a gold inlay, and most of these are to provide protection for weakened tooth structure. Therefore the cavity design for small gold inlays is of only limited practical importance, but inlays still have a role to play for larger restorations protecting the tooth.

PRINCIPLES OF CAVITY DESIGN

A number of stages are suggested for designing cavities. These are a sequence of practical steps and thought processes. Part of the clinician's role is to make judgements (see Chapter 2), and this must be done throughout the procedure rather than making a single decision at the beginning and then following it slavishly. In the case of a carious tooth the stages will often be as follows:

- gain access to the caries

- remove the caries

- put the instruments down, look, think, and design

- complete the preparation.

Gaining access to the caries

The relatively small carious lesion, which nevertheless needs to be restored, presents a problem of access when it is on the occlusal surface, the approximal surface, or around and beneath existing restorations. Access is not usually a problem with initial lesions on the buccal and lingual surfaces of teeth.

Access to caries in the occlusal dentine is made by cutting through the overlying enamel. With more advanced lesions this undermined enamel will already have caved in, opening up immediate access to the carious dentine.

There are at least four ways of gaining access to caries on the approximal surface of a posterior tooth (Fig. 3.3). When the lesion is sufficiently large that it is inevitable that the marginal ridge will have to be removed, access is gained just inside the marginal ridge and the remainder of the marginal ridge is broken away shortly afterwards. The marginal ridge is not cut directly, as this would almost inevitably cause damage to the adjacent tooth. The second method is to gain access via buccal or lingual surfaces. This is more appropriate where there is a distorted contact point producing caries towards the gingival end of the approximal surface, leaving a sound marginal ridge. It is more practical where there has been a degree of gingival recession. The third method is to approach from the occlusal surface, leaving the marginal ridge intact. Fourthly, when the adjacent tooth has been extracted for other reasons, direct access is possible. However, in many cases removing the adjacent tooth will improve access for cleaning, and even relatively large enamel lesions will partially remineralize and arrest so that restoration may not be necessary.

Access to the approximal surfaces of anterior teeth with minimal lesions is usually from the lingual or palatal surface, leaving as much of the intact buccal enamel as possible, even though it may be unsupported by dentine. On occasions, for example with overlapping teeth, buccal or even incisal access is more sensible (see Fig. 9.2).

Gaining access to caries around existing restorations can be the most difficult of these procedures. When the whole restoration has to be removed then the problem is relatively straightforward, but increasingly the virtues of repairing existing amalgam or composite restorations are being acknowledged. For this reason access to caries is usually at the expense of part of the restoration, rather than sound

Fig. 3.3 Access can be gained to approximal caries in one of four ways (see text).

enamel, but without destroying the retention and other characteristics of the restoration. If the operator is not confident that all the caries has been reached it is safer to remove the whole of the old restoration. Chapter 11 describes why it is sometimes better to leave part of the old restoration in place.

Removing the caries

Once sufficient access is available, caries is removed from the enamel–dentine junction. Caries should not be left at the enamel–dentine junction because no restorative material forms a perfect cavity seal and the disease may progress more readily if caries is left in this area. In addition, enamel undermined by caries is vulnerable to fracture in areas of occlusal stress.

It is not always easy to judge when the enamel–dentine junction is caries-free. Traditionally, the aim has been to remove all *demineralized* tissue in this area. To this end cavity preparation continues until the enamel–dentine junction looks stain-free and feels hard to a sharp probe. However, recent work has shown that areas of hard but stained dentine at the enamel–dentine junction may be as minimally infected as adjacent stain-free areas. Thus, the authors are forced to question whether the enamel–dentine junction should be made stain-free as well as hard. Certainly, where tooth tissue is at a premium, the authors currently 'break the rules' and leave stained but hard tissue at the enamel–dentine junction.

The final stage in caries removal is to deal with the dentine over the pulp. Since demineralization precedes bacterial penetration, the interface between the dentine that is demineralized and that which is infected would be an ideal place to stop tissue removal. This is the rationale behind the technique of *indirect pulp capping*, when stained but firm dentine is left in the base of a cavity in a symptomless vital tooth to avoid exposure. The demineralized dentine which remains is then covered with a therapeutic material (usually calcium hydroxide) to encourage reparative dentine formation and remineralization of residual dentine, and to kill any remaining micro-organisms.

The problem for the clinician is to distinguish between the dentine which should be removed and that which may be left. Currently, clinical judgement is used to make this decision and the best rule of thumb is that the soft dentine is heavily infected and should therefore be removed.

Research indicates that it may be important to isolate a deep cavity from saliva, since it has been shown that micro-exposures (a pulpal exposure that is too small to see) will often heal by reparative dentine formation provided that bacterial contamination is minimized. For this reason, a rubber dam (see p. 79) is helpful when restoring very carious teeth.

Where excavation of pulpal caries results in an obvious carious exposure, removal of the pulp and root canal therapy is usually necessary if the tooth is to be saved. Occasionally, a small carious exposure in an otherwise symptomless and vital tooth may be dressed with calcium hydroxide. This *direct pulp cap* aims to preserve a healthy vital pulp by encouraging dentine bridge formation to wall off the exposure.

Put the instruments down: look, think, and design.

This is the most important stage in the preparation. Poor decisions lead to as many failures as poor technique. The main decisions to be made are as follows:

- the final choice of restorative material

- how to retain the restorative material in the cavity

- design features to protect the remaining tooth tissue

- design features to optimize the strength of the restoration
- the shape and position of the cavity margin.

The final choice of restorative material

In most cases the cavity will be started with the expectation of using a particular material, and in most cases this decision is obvious from the outset and is not altered at this stage. However, in other cavities the extent of the caries will be greater or less than was anticipated and a change of plan may be necessary. For instance, if the caries was more extensive than anticipated, a decision to restore with amalgam may be altered to the choice of an inlay with cuspal protection. Alternatively, the adhesive materials, glass ionomer cement and composite resin, may be used to reinforce weakened dentine and enamel. Similarly, with occlusal caries, a decision may be made at this stage between an amalgam restoration, composite restoration, or a combined composite restoration and fissure sealant.

Making the preparation retentive

Retention can be defined as the features of a preparation which prevent the restoration falling out in any direction. Retention for any restoration should be visualized as preventing loss of the restoration in five directions (Fig. 3.4):

- occlusally
- buccally
- lingually/palatally
- mesially
- distally

or at angles between these directions.

In an amalgam restoration which restores two surfaces of the tooth, say the occlusal and buccal surfaces, features will be required which prevent the loss of the restoration occlusally and buccally. With a large restoration, retention will be required in three, four, or even all five directions.

The means by which the restorative material will be retained permanently within the cavity vary according to the material. Amalgam needs to be retained by physical means, such as undercuts in the preparation, retention grooves, and pins. Each part of the amalgam cavity should be independently retentive. Thus, with the occlusal–buccal or palatal restoration, it is ideal if both the occlusal and buccal or palatal parts are retentive independently of each other (Fig. 3.5).

Composite restorations are attached to enamel by acid etching, which produces a large number of small retentive pores into which the resin flows. It is still a mechanical form of retention relying on these miniature undercut cavities and is sometimes referred to as micromechanical retention (Fig. 3.6). Retention of composite to dentine may be achieved by mechanical undercuts or by using a dentine bonding agent or by an intermediate layer of glass ionomer cement (see Chapter 8, p. 141).

Glass ionomer cement bonds adequately to enamel and dentine by chemical means and does not require mechanical undercuts unless subjected to occlusal forces.

Cast gold and other alloy restorations are retained by means of a different type of micromechanical retention with the gold surface and the prepared tooth surface interlocked with rigid cement (Fig. 3.7). For this reason the path of insertion of the restoration must be within the angle shown in Fig. 3.7 and described in more detail in Chapter 10.

Fig. 3.4 Cavities should be designed with retentive features which prevent the restoration being lost in all five directions and at any angle between them.

Fig. 3.5 An occlusal–palatal cavity, both parts of which are independently retentive.

Fig. 3.6   Fig. 3.7

Fig. 3.6 A scanning electron micrograph of etched enamel. Field width, 20 μm. (Reproduced by courtesy of Dr M. O. Atta.)

Fig. 3.7 A scanning electron micrograph of a dentine–cement–cast metal interface. The cement, in this case, is not adhesive and so the surfaces can separate at the angle shown. However, if they are to separate at angles less than this, the areas of cement within the irregularities of the metal or dentine surface would need to shear and crumble away. Field width, 100 μm. (Reproduced by courtesy of Dr M. O. Atta.)

Design features to protect the remaining tooth tissue

The remaining tooth tissue, particularly the enamel, may be vulnerable to fracture as a result of either occlusal forces or the insertion of a restoration.

With amalgam restorations, unsupported enamel on the occlusal surface should be removed, as should sharp edges of enamel elsewhere. Although these latter edges are not vulnerable to occlusal forces, they may be damaged in tightening a metal matrix band or while condensing the amalgam (see Chapter 7).

It is less important to remove undermined enamel when etched composite restorations are used, because the composite will support the enamel except in areas subjected to direct occlusal forces. Articulating paper should be used to check the exact contact areas between opposing teeth to help with the decision as to whether or not to remove unsupported occlusal enamel.

When the cavity is large and the remaining cusps are weak, the choice is to remove the weak cusp altogether, to protect it from occlusal forces by covering its occlusal surface by means of a cast metal inlay/onlay, or to support it by bonding it to other parts of the tooth with glass ionomer cement, composite resin, or a combination of the two materials (see Chapters 7 and 10).

Design features to optimize the strength of the restoration

Some restorative materials, particularly amalgam and porcelain, are weak in thin sections and when they have sharp angles. This means that sufficient tooth tissue should be removed to allow adequate thickness of the material. In addition, cavo-surface angles of amalgam and porcelain preparations should approximate to 90 degrees to allow sufficient bulk of material at the margin.

A good example of this design feature is in the occlusal–proximal amalgam restoration in which the angle between the occlusal floor and axial wall of the preparation is rounded over or bevelled. This is done because the amalgam in this region is shallow, since there is usually an occlusal fossa immediately above it. This area coincides with the narrowest part of the occlusal preparation and a cavity with a sharp internal angle would concentrate stresses, increasing the likelihood of the amalgam fracturing here (Fig. 3.8).

Fig. 3.8 The proximal box of an occlusal–proximal amalgam cavity. The angle between the occlusal floor and axial wall of the box has been bevelled (B) for the reasons described in the text. Note also that the corners of the box are also rounded (A) to reduce the risk of voids in the amalgam here, resulting from the difficulty in packing amalgam into sharp angles.

'Resistance form'

In older terminology relating to stylized cavity shapes and originating with G.V. Black, 'retention form' was a term used to describe the design features of a cavity which prevented loss of the restoration axially. 'Resistance form' was used to describe design features which resisted loss in other directions. This distinction is no longer useful, in particular in relation to the retention mechanisms of acid etching. Therefore the term 'retention' should be used as it is described on p. 60, and the term 'resistance', if it is needed at all, should now be applied to the design features described in the two previous paragraphs.

The shape and position of the cavity margin

The shape of the cavity margin will largely be determined by the choice of material. Amalgam and porcelain cavity margins should be finished at approximately 90 degrees as described earlier. Cast metal restorations can be finished to acute angles, and so the cavity margin can be a very oblique bevel. The shape of the margin for composite restorations may be bevelled in some cases to improve retention and appearance (see Chapters 6 and 8).

Cavity margins should be supragingival wherever possible to improve access for cleaning. In posterior restorations involving the approximal surface, a decision must be made as to whether or not the margin of the preparations should be extended beyond the contact area to improve access for cleaning. Traditionally, it has always been cut clear of the contact area, but this is no longer considered necessary, particularly with glass ionomer cement restorations. Cutting the cavity free of the contact area may well be more destructive than is necessary in a number of cases (see Chapter 7).

With anterior approximal restorations the cavity margin is commonly left in contact with the adjacent teeth for aesthetic reasons and because access for cleaning is good anteriorly.

POSSIBLE FUTURE DEVELOPMENTS IN CAVITY DESIGN

Looking back at the changes which have occurred in the approach to cavity design in the last 30 years, it is inevitable that further changes will occur in the future. Therefore the principles outlined above should be regarded as the current 'state of play' and not set in concrete in the dentist's mind.

It is possible that we are at the threshold of a major development in thinking about restoring teeth. Until now the concept has been to remove diseased hard tissue and replace it with little more than a plug in a hole. (Fillings used to be known as 'stoppings'.) The only materials available until fairly recently had very little resemblance—structurally, chemically, aesthetically, or functionally—to dental tissues. They did not bond adequately to the dental tissues and (with the exception of silicate cement) did not have therapeutic properties such as resisting recurrent caries. Despite these drawbacks they served their purpose adequately. However, new objectives are emerging. In the future the emphasis will be more on genuinely *restoring* teeth rather than just repairing them. One example of this approach is the remineralization of early enamel lesions rather than cutting out the diseased tissue. Another example is the 'layered' restoration in which a cavity is filled with glass ionomer cement (or cermet) to replace the dentine and then is 'topped off' with a layer of composite to replace the enamel. The properties of glass ionomer cement are nearer to those of dentine than they are to enamel, and the material bonds to dentine and leaches fluoride. The composite, which can be attached micromechanically to the surface of the glass ionomer cement and the etched enamel walls, replaces the enamel and has a similar appearance. Its properties resemble enamel more than glass ionomer cement does. This 'layered' restoration is not yet a true reconstruction of the tooth, but it is closer than a restoration in amalgam.

In the future these attempts may be seen as the crude start to a new era in which cavity design may be drastically altered or indeed become unnecessary, either because new techniques or new materials become available. Many anterior restorations needed for reasons of trauma, toothwear, or hypoplasia already require little cavity preparation other than acid etching or chemical bonding.

THE CONTROL OF PAIN AND TRAUMA IN OPERATIVE DENTISTRY

Some operative procedures are painless, some are uncomfortable, and many are potentially painful. It is not sufficient simply to give a local anaesthetic; many procedures can still be uncomfortable, for example heavy-handed lip retraction, trapping the lip between the teeth and an instrument, and requiring a tense patient to keep his/her mouth open for long periods without relaxing. All these are sufficiently uncomfortable to deter many patients from visiting the dentist even when pulpal anaesthesia is effective. Patients should not be expected to submit to anything more than minor discomfort of short duration, unless the measures required to avoid it would require greater discomfort or risk to their general well-being.

Pre-operative precautions

Proper diagnosis of the condition of the pulp before administering local anaesthesia is necessary. Sometimes local anaesthesia has been provided without establishing the condition of the pulp, only to find later that the tooth was root-filled or contained a necrotic pulp.

Some patients, particularly later in life, have formed sufficient secondary dentine for their teeth to be insensitive to all but the most extensive preparation. These patients may not need local anaesthesia. However, for the majority of patients local anaesthesia is required once it is established that the pulp is vital. It is bad practice to leave administration of a local anaesthetic until it is essential because the patient is experiencing pain. This is unpleasant for the patient and destroys confidence.

Alternative or additional methods of controlling pain and apprehension are relative analgesia with nitrous oxide–oxygen mixtures in conjunction with local anaesthetics, oral or intravenous sedation with midazolam or diazepam, or in some cases full general anaesthesia. These methods are only very rarely required if the patient is handled sympathetically and gently. Some patients who have had a traumatic dental experience or need a difficult form of treatment may be offered one of these approaches but, where possible, they should be weaned off it again as soon as possible in their own interest. There are two reasons for this. First, if elaborate precautions such as these need to be taken, dental treatment tends to be deferred until batches of treatment are necessary and this is not the best way to maintain a healthy dentition. Second, as was stressed in Chapter 1, effective communication between operator and patient is necessary if the patient is to co-operate in all the preventive measures necessary for long-term dental health. This is not possible with a sedated or unconscious patient.

Pain and trauma control during tooth preparation

Patients usually prefer the airotor to preparation of teeth at low speed because of the vibration felt at low speed (see Chapter 5). This vibration can be minimized by ensuring that the handpiece bearings are in good condition and by deadening the vibration by pressure on the tooth with a finger while it is being prepared. This vibration should not deter the operator from completing the removal of caries at low speed, because using the airotor will almost inevitably result in unnecessary tooth destruction.

With an anaesthetized tooth there is a danger of causing thermal damage to the pulp by inadequate cooling of the bur. Figure 3.9(a) shows the pulp immediately below a very deep cavity cut at low speed under a continuous stream of water; the tooth was extracted shortly afterwards. Here the pulp shows no detectable signs of injury. Figure 3.9(b), in contrast, shows the pulp condition 11 days after using a high-speed handpiece without water spray. The destruction of the odontoblast layer is clearly seen, with all the cellular and vascular changes of inflammation.

(a)

(b)

Fig. 3.9   (a) Pulp below the deepest part of a cavity prepared at 5000 rev/minute under a constant stream of water.
(b) Localized destructive lesion of the pulp adjacent to a cavity prepared with an airotor without water spray. (Reproduced by courtesy of Professor D. S. Shovelton.)

Direct trauma to the pulp should of course be avoided, although probably all dentists have occasionally exposed pulp at the base of a deep cavity when they were not expecting to. This may be because the pulp is unusually large or has not formed reparative dentine at the rate which would normally be expected. The terms 'carious exposure' and 'traumatic exposure' are used to describe exposure of a vital bleeding pulp. The distinction between the two is not always clear, but in the former the dentist feels that exposure is inevitable if all the soft dentine is removed whereas in the latter it is not.

Direct trauma to the gingival tissues should be avoided, and careful selection of the size of bur to be used, adequate support of the handpiece, and a gentle technique will usually prevent this. Occasionally, with cavities that extend well below the gingival margin, it is necessary to retract the gingival tissues with a rubber dam or to remove gingival tissue surgically.

Avoiding post-operative pain

Post-operative pain may arise from the lips and soft tissues if they have been stretched or damaged. It may also arise from the pulp if it has been damaged or the cavity has been inadequately lined. Finally, pain may come from the periapical periodontal tissues if the restoration is left high so that the tooth is in traumatic occlusion. These circumstances should all be avoided.

CAVITY LINING AND CHEMICAL PREPARATION

A whole battery of materials are now available for the treatment of a prepared cavity surface. These materials include the following:

- Linings, such as calcium hydroxide and glass ionomer cement, are placed on a cavity floor for protective, therapeutic, or structural reasons.

- Varnishes, which are natural or synthetic resins in a solvent, are applied to cavity walls in an attempt to improve the marginal seal of an amalgam restoration.

- Etchants, which are phosphoric acid solutions or gels, are used to create porosities in enamel to facilitate mechanical adhesion of resin restorative materials.

- Dentine bonding agents are used to facilitate physico-chemical adhesion of composites to dentine.

- Conditioners, which are weak acids, are used to remove organic debris before placing a glass ionomer cement that is chemically adhesive to enamel and dentine.

A dental materials textbook should be consulted for details of the chemical composition and setting reactions of these materials.

Objectives and materials

The objectives in preparing a cavity to receive a restorative material can be considered under the following headings:

- cleaning the cavity

- therapeutic

- protective

- structural

- attaining cavity seal and promoting adhesion.

These objectives will be discussed below, together with the materials currently available. The clinical techniques for handling the materials will be found in Part II of this book.

Cleaning the cavity

Cavity preparation, without water spray, produces grinding debris and it is important to wash the cavity thoroughly to remove this. Before placing the restorative material the cavity should be dried with air.

Therapeutic

Cavity preparation is usually carried out to remove dental caries. Details of the management of carious dentine have been given on p. 59. A therapeutic lining material is placed on the partly demineralized dentine in the base of the cavity for the following reasons:

- to stimulate the odontoblasts to lay down reparative dentine

- to encourage remineralization of the dentine

- to kill any bacteria that may remain in the base of the cavity.

The preferred material in these circumstances is a setting cement containing calcium hydroxide, which is believed to achieve each of these objectives. It is believed that, to be effective, the calcium hydroxide must be released from the cement. The material should be used as a thin layer for its therapeutic effect and then covered with glass ionomer cement if further thermal insulation is required.

Antibiotic-corticosteroid preparations have also been used as therapeutic lining materials. These preparations are unrivalled in their ability to suppress the pain of pulpitis when placed on carious exposures. Unfortunately, their use is a temporary expedient, since pulp death almost invariably occurs some time later. For this reason they should only be used where root canal treatment is planned and insufficient time or inadequate anaesthesia prevent pulp extirpation at that visit.

Protective

Thermal

If the cavity is to be filled with amalgam or cast metal an insulating layer may be required between the metal filling and the pulp-dentine complex. Fortunately, dentine itself is a good insulator and thus there is no justification for removing it to make room for an insulating layer. However, in a deep or moderately deep cavity there may be insufficient thickness of dentine remaining and the cavity will then require a lining.

A glass ionomer cement is a good choice but must be sublined with calcium hydroxide in deep cavities. However, it bonds to the dentine walls and releases fluoride, and it can be used in much thicker layers than other lining materials. If the restoration is to be amalgam, the glass ionomer lining should be designed so that the amalgam is thick enough for strength. If composite is to be used the glass ionomer cement lining is usually built up to the enamel–dentine junction (or overbuilt and cut back to this level when set). In other words, the glass ionomer cement replaces all the dentine and the composite replaces the enamel.

Chemical

The pulp-dentine complex may require protection from restorative materials, such as composite resin, that are thought to be toxic. It is not entirely clear why composite resins are potentially damaging to a vital pulp; one obvious explanation is that they may be cytotoxic to the odontoblasts. However, the fact that the materials do not seal the cavity adequately seems to be more important, since micro-organisms can thus pass between the filling and the cavity wall and cause a pulpal reaction. For these reasons the dentine is protected with a lining, and composites are placed against etched cavity walls to minimize leakage. The recommended base for composites or glass ionomer materials is a setting cement containing calcium hydroxide.

Structural

It is possible to use a lining material to restore the internal form of a cavity (see p. 170) to produce a flat pulpal floor and a smooth axial wall. This means that less filling material will be required and the internal shape of the cavity may be less complex. Both these factors are of considerable advantage when using cast metal as an intracoronal restoration. A glass ionomer cement is an ideal material for this purpose because it has a cariostatic effect due to the fluoride that it contains. It is also adhesive to dentine and thus may afford some support to the weakened tooth tissue.

Attaining cavity seal and promoting adhesion

If a filling does not seal a cavity, leakage of bacteria and fluids carrying molecules and ions in solution can occur between the restoration and the cavity wall. Such leakage may result in recurrent caries, tooth discoloration under amalgams, hypersensitivity, pulpal damage, and a rapid breakdown of certain filling materials. All restorative materials leak to some extent but there is much that can be done to improve cavity seal.

Amalgam

Amalgam is neither chemically nor mechanically adhesive to enamel and dentine; it merely fills the hole. The freshly packed amalgam restoration leaks, although with time the seal improves, probably because corrosion products from the filling material block the space between the amalgam and the cavity wall. However, several laboratory studies have shown that the initial seal of the restoration can be improved by painting the cavity walls with a proprietary cavity varnish before placing the filling. All varnishes currently available are soluble to some extent but it is hoped that corrosion products of the amalgam will fill the space occupied by the varnish as it dissolves away.

Composite resin and glass ionomer cement

Acid etching of enamel cavity walls with phosphoric acid prior to placing a composite resin creates porosities in the enamel. An unfilled bonding resin is then applied which flows into these microspaces to form resin tags which physically retain the composite restoration. The acid etch technique improves the marginal seal of the material. However, there is considerable argument as to whether cavity margins should be bevelled to improve the bond.

Many attempts have been made to develop intermediate adhesive systems capable of bonding composite restorations to dentine. One obstacle to achieving this is the wetness of cut dentine. Another problem is shrinkage of the composite material as it polymerizes. In a cavity bounded by both enamel and dentine the bond to acid-etched enamel will be stronger than the bond to dentine. A material that shrinks as it sets will move towards the stronger bond, leaving a potential gap between restoration and tooth on the dentine side of the cavity. This gap is at the cervical margin of the restoration in an area of plaque stagnation and is thus particularly prone to recurrent caries.

Currently there are four approaches to obtaining a reliable bond between the restoration and the dentine.

Resin composites and dentine bonding agents. Modern dentine bonding agents may overcome the problems of polymerization shrinkage of the resin. It is claimed that these agents rapidly achieve a high dentine bond strength which will resist the contraction of the resin material towards the bond with acid-etched enamel.

The surface of cut dentine is wet, is less mineralized than enamel, and consists of a smear layer of adherent amorphous calcific debris produced by the action of any cutting instrument. Dentine bonding agents have been developed to adhere to dentine via the smear layer. Alternatively, the smear layer is modified or totally removed. The exposed dentine is then infiltrated with the resin.

The smear layer is completely or partially removed with weak acid. The water-repellent (hydrophobic) resin is now required to stick to a watery substrate. To overcome this problem, a volatile low-molecular-weight hydrophilic primer is now placed over the altered surface of the dentine. This flows into the dentinal tubules and intertubular dentine between them, retaining the bonding agent micromechanically and acting as a 'wetting agent' for succeeding layers. These layers are less hydrophilic and have a higher molecular weight, and they are polymerized either by self curing or light curing. This embodies the dentine in an increasingly hydrophobic and stiff material which is then available to bond to any composite placed over it (Fig. 3.10).

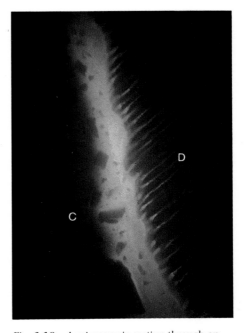

Fig. 3.10 A microscopic section through an adhesive interface. The dentine bonding agent flows into the dentinal tubules (D), mechanically locking into them and so retaining the restoration (C). This image was obtained using a scanning optical microscope with the various components of the adhesive labelled with dyes. The composite restoration is on the left and the dentine is on the right. (Reproduced by courtesy of *The British Dental Journal*.)

Conventional glass ionomer cements.   These materials are one of the most exciting developments in dentistry; they are the first practical tooth-coloured chemically adhesive restorative materials. Glass ionomers bond dynamically to both dentine and enamel by ionic exchange at the interface of the mineralized tissue and the cement. Their adhesion is less than that achieved by the resin-based materials, but the adhesive interface is capable of limited self-repair. Modern materials have a good appearance and improved physical properties, although translucency is still difficult to achieve. To obtain clinically reliable bond strengths a clean dry tooth surface is necessary. Weak concentrations of polyacrylic acid are applied to remove surface debris and the superficial smear layer from the dentine, thus providing a clean surface for bonding.

Layered technique.   Lost dentine is replaced with glass ionomer cement and enamel is replaced by a composite resin. There is controversy over the need to etch the glass ionomer prior to placing the composite. Etching times in excess of 15 seconds may reduce the bond strength between the two materials.

Resin-modified glass ionomer cements.   These materials are relatively new. They are easy to handle because the set of the resin component of the material is initiated by light curing. Although they may shrink as they set, expansion due to water uptake by the resin may compensate for the initial resin shrinkage. When these materials are used in a layered technique they should chemically bond to the resin composite without the need for etching.

FURTHER READING

Eley, B. M. and Cox, S. W. (1993). The release, absorption and possible health effects of mercury from dental amalgam: a review of recent findings. *Br. Dent. J.* **175**, 355–62.

Kidd, E. A. M. and Joyston-Bechal, S. (1996). The operative management of caries. *Essentials of dental caries*, Chapter 11. Oxford Medical Publications, Oxford.

Kidd, E. A. M., Joyston-Bechal, S., and Beighton, D. (1993). Microbiological validation of assessment of caries activity during cavity preparation. *Caries Res.* **27**, 402–8.

Mount, G. J. (1994). *An atlas of glass-ionomer cements. A clinician's guide.* Martin Dunitz, London.

Phillips, R. W. (1991). *Skinner's science of dental materials.* W. B. Saunders, Philadelphia, PA.

Smith, B. G. N., Wright, P. S., and Brown, D. (1994). *The clinical handling of dental materials.* John Wright, Bristol.

Watson, T. F. and Bartlett, D. W. (1994). Adhesive systems: composites, dentine bonding agents and glass ionomers. *Br. Dent. J.* **176**, 227–31.

PART II

TREATMENT TECHNIQUES

4 The operator and the environment

THE DENTAL TEAM

Dentists are leaders of a group of individuals whose combined efforts are devoted to the restoration and preservation of dental health. The dentist is assisted at the chairside by a dental nurse, sometimes called a dental surgery assistant (DSA). Many dentists employ hygienists to whom they delegate some of the preventive aspects of dental care such as oral hygiene instruction, scaling and polishing, dietary advice, and fluoride application. Technical work, such as making crowns and dentures, is carried out to the dentist's prescription by a dental technician who may work in a laboratory attached to the practice or in a separate commercial laboratory. These members of the team, who are all directly or indirectly involved in providing dental care, will usually have appropriate qualifications (in the case of hygienists they *must* be qualified). In addition, most dentists employ receptionists, secretaries, practice managers, or some combination of such team members who do not need a special dental qualification.

The dental student should meet and work with all groups of clinical ancillary personnel from the beginning of clinical training if at all possible. Such contact is an important part of training because it develops effective communication with them and a proper understanding of their roles which is essential to the smooth running of the dental team.

THE DENTAL SCHOOL AND PRACTICE ENVIRONMENT

The dental school environment is obviously very different from general practice, although many features are common to both. There is an entrance, which should be well signposted so that the patient knows where to go and is not embarrassed by finding himself/herself in the doctor's surgery next door or in the wrong hospital department. Other information, such as hours of opening and arrangements for out-of-hours emergency treatment, should be clearly but discreetly shown.

Everyone concerned with dental care should appreciate that the hospital or practice, which seems so commonplace when one works in it every day, is a new and possibly frightening environment for patients. Dentists and staff should look critically at the surroundings to see that they are as attractive and welcoming as possible. Design, decor, and cleanliness are important; plants and magazines in a waiting area are a welcoming sight. Even more important is the personal touch: a friendly smile from the receptionist and the prompt attention of the dentist or student, or a genuine apology for unavoidable delay, all help to transform what is often a worrying experience for patients into a warm and welcoming one.

THE SURGERY

Positioning the patient, the dentist, and the dental nurse

Patient, dentist, and dental nurse must all be positioned for maximum comfort and visibility, with minimum distortion of backs and necks. Initially, the dentist and patient need to talk to each other, and this should be with both seated face to face on the same level (Fig. 4.1). If the dentist stands towering over the patient or talks to the back of his or her head, communication is poor and the patient feels even more at a disadvantage.

Figure 4.1   Dentist and patient talking.

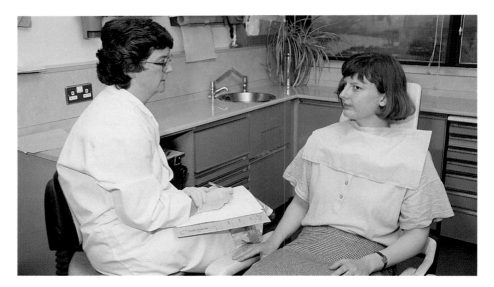

When the time comes to examine the patient, or perform operative treatment, the dental chair is tilted back and raised so that the patient is horizontal (Fig. 4.2). The chair should be designed to support the patient's head, back, and arms. The patient's head should be at the top of the head-rest, so that the dentist does not have to bend forward excessively to see into the mouth, and at the dentist's mid-sternum level bringing the mouth to the correct focal range of the eyes. The dentist's knees will now fit under the head-rest.

Figure 4.2   Dentist, dental nurse, and patient positioned to carry out an intraoral examination. Note that the patient has now been provided with eye protection. Once the dentist starts to operate, the dental nurse should also wear protective spectacles.

The dentist sits, usually behind the patient, on a chair with castor feet which enable it to be moved easily by the operator while seated. The dentist's back is supported, feet flat on the floor and the top of the thighs sloping about 15 degrees to the horizontal. The long axis of the dentist's upper arm should be vertical and the elbows close to the rib cage, while the head is tilted forward so that the eyes can see the fingertips.

For a right-handed dentist, the dental nurse sits on the patient's left-hand side, facing the patient. Her chair should also have a back-rest, but for her to be able to see clearly into the mouth she should be seated some 10 cm (4 inches) higher than the dentist; thus her chair may require a bar on which she can rest her feet (Fig. 4.2).

So far, the vertical positioning of the dentist's chair, the dental chair, and the dental nurse's chair have been considered. Positioning must also be considered in a horizontal plane. If the patient's head in the dental chair is represented by a clock-face, the dentist usually sits slightly to the right-hand side of the patient, at 11 o'clock, but with the facility to move between 1 and 8 o'clock. The dental nurse is usually positioned at 4 o'clock, but may also take up a position anywhere between 1 o'clock and 4 o'clock (Fig. 4.2).

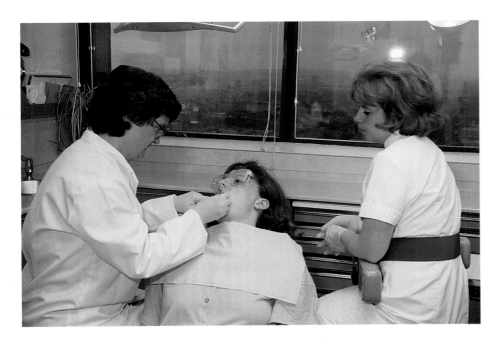

Fig. 4.3 Dentist in the 8 o'clock position examining the lower right quadrant by direct vision.

The patient may also be asked to turn his or her head towards or away from the dentist. For example, when examining the buccal surfaces of teeth in the upper left quadrant the patient's head should be turned to the right so that this area can be seen clearly by direct vision.

Although the dentist usually sits at 11 o'clock, some operators move round to the 8 o'clock position and readjust the patient's chair when working on the lower right quadrant by direct vision. The base of the chair should be lowered and the back-rest raised slightly, the patient's head turned towards the dentist (Fig. 4.3).

Unfortunately, much dental equipment is designed for right-handed dentists and is not readily adapted for left-handed use. Much of this advice on positioning will not apply to left-handed dentists, and their position will not simply be the reverse of the right-handed dentist's position because of the inflexibility of the equipment. Left-handed dentists usually need to experiment with positions until they are able to equip a surgery for their own use.

Lighting

If the dentist is to see well, the small operating field must be lit adequately. The level of illumination of the surgery as a whole, whether by natural or artificial light, should be bright and is usually above that needed for normal purposes so that there is not too much contrast with the higher level of illumination of the operating field. This reduces the extent to which the dentist's and dental nurse's eyes have to adapt. The operating light is situated above the patient's head and its direction is varied with the arch being examined. Auxiliary means of intra-oral illumination will be discussed in Chapter 5, p. 103.

Siting of work-surfaces and instruments

The dentist and dental nurse need work-surfaces around them on which to place instruments and materials. The dental nurse needs facilities for mixing materials, and the dentist needs an area for the patient's notes and a viewing box for radiographs.

The dentist requires easy access to the handpieces and hand instruments. These may be situated on the dentist's side of the chair, above the patient's chest, or on the dental nurse's side of the chair (Fig. 4.4). Each of these positions has disadvantages. The dental nurse cannot reach the instruments if they are on the dentist's side and therefore has to walk around the chair at least once between each patient. Many patients feel claustrophobic with instruments and trays positioned over their chest.

(a)

(b)

Fig. 4.4 (a) Instruments on the dentist's side of the chair.
(b) Instruments on the cervical tray over the patient's chest.
(c) Instruments on the dental nurse's side of the chair.

(c)

When handpieces and instruments are on the dental nurse's side this layout also presupposes that she will always be present to pass them to the dentist. A fourth possibility—the instruments placed behind the head of the chair—has the major disadvantage that it increases the risk that instruments will be passed over the patient's face and dropped, causing injury. This possibility, together with the awkwardness of the instruments being behind the dentist's back, makes this the least popular arrangement.

It is obvious that surgery design, even for a single dentist, is open to considerable variation. In a dental school, where operating areas must be designed for right- and left-handed students working with and without dental nurses, the problems are virtually insoluble. Maximum flexibility must be allowed with work-surfaces provided on both sides, and this is also important in a dental practice where the dentist may have to work unaided for limited periods.

Aspirating equipment; cavity washing and drying

High-speed cutting instruments require water cooling, and cavities must be washed, dried, and isolated from saliva. Thus, suction equipment to remove liquids from the mouth is essential, as is a syringe which will deliver a jet of water or air, or a spray mixture of the two—a three-in-one syringe. Aspiration of liquids and cavity washing and drying should be a principal responsibility of the dental nurse and so the equipment must be available on her side of the chair. In addition, a three-in-one syringe should also be available on the dentist's side to allow the operator to work alone if necessary. At the end of treatment patients like to rinse their mouths, and a spittoon is commonly available on the dental nurse's side of the chair. An alternative is a large funnel, which can be autoclaved, attached to a suction tube as shown in Fig. 4.4 (c).

Hand and instrument cleaning

Handbasins should be available to both dentist and dental nurse. Instrument cleaning and sterilizing facilities should be on the dental nurse's side of the surgery, when not provided centrally in a hospital. It is the dentist's responsibility to ensure sterility and clean working practices (see Chapter 5).

CLOSE-SUPPORT DENTISTRY

Close-support or four-handed dentistry are the terms used to describe systems of close co-operation between dentist and dental nurse in the actual dental treatment of patients. Such co-operation is essential for maximum operating effectiveness. Unfortunately, many dental students spend a major part of their course operating alone, and acquire time-wasting and inefficient operating habits which then have to be corrected if their clinical standards are not to fall when they enter the hurly-burly of general practice. Fortunately, some four-handed dentistry is now taught in dental schools, and it is important that students learn how a trained and efficient dental nurse works so that they can subsequently train an assistant to work with them happily and efficiently.

Maintaining a clear working field for the dentist

A principal duty of the dental nurse in close-support dentistry is to maintain a clear working field so that the patient is comfortable and the dentist can see the working area. This involves aspiration of water and coolant spray, retraction of soft tissues, keeping the mirror free of spray, and keeping the cavity clear of debris.

When aspirating, the dental nurse should place the aspirator in the mouth *before* the dentist positions the mirror and handpiece. She first retracts the lip with her finger or the tip of the three-in-one syringe and then places the aspirator tip in position (Fig. 4.5(a)). The dentist may then position the mirror and handpiece (Fig. 4.5(b)). If this order is reversed the dentist's view is likely to be obstructed by the aspirator tip, and for the same reason the aspirator should not cross the arch on which the dentist is working. The tip of the aspirator should never contact the patient's soft palate as this might cause retching.

(a)   (b)   (c)

Fig. 4.5 (a) Dental nurse retracting the patient's lip and placing the aspirator tip next to the tooth to be prepared.
(b) Once the aspirator tip is in position, the dentist may position the mirror and the handpiece.
(c) An alternative position for the aspirator tip is just distal to the last molar which is where water will naturally collect with the patient supine.

The orifice of the aspirator tip may be positioned either 'on site' (Fig. 4.5(a)) or retromolar (Fig. 4.5(c)). In either position the aspirator tip also retracts soft tissue. When 'on site' it is placed next to the tooth being prepared, level with its occlusal plane on the side of the arch nearest to the dental nurse. The bevel of the aspirator tip is parallel to the arch and about 1 cm away from the tooth so that the coolant spray is not diverted away from the tooth. Alternatively, the aspirator tip can be placed 'retromolar', just distal to the last molar, which is where water will naturally collect with the patient supine.

The dental nurse also assists with soft tissue retraction in other ways, mainly with tissues on her side of the arch. Thus, when working on the left side of the mouth, the cheek and lips on the patient's left side are the responsibility of the dental nurse, whilst tongue retraction is the responsibility of the dentist. Conversely, when working on the right-hand side, tongue retraction is the responsibility of the dental nurse while the dentist retracts lips and cheeks.

When cutting with the airotor, the mirror surface quickly becomes obscured by spray. The dental nurse should keep the mirror clear by washing it with spray and blowing air over it (Fig. 4.6). Each time the cutting stops, the dental nurse should wash and dry the cavity and the mirror so that the dentist can see clearly.

Instrument transfer

Fig. 4.6 The dental nurse is using a three-in-one syringe to wash and dry the mirror while the dentist uses the airotor.

In efficient close-support dentistry all hand instruments are on a work surface in front of the dental nurse, who hands them to the dentist. This means that the dentist can concentrate on the mouth at all times without having repeatedly to look away to pick up and replace instruments. However, if dentist and dental nurse are going to work efficiently, the dentist must use a fixed sequence of instruments for any procedure and the dental nurse must anticipate which instrument the dentist will require next.

When passing an instrument the dental nurse picks it up at its non-working end (Fig. 4.7(a)), leaving sufficient length of instrument shaft for the dentist.

Instruments to be passed to the dentist's right hand are picked up with the dental nurse's left hand. The dental nurse would only pass a mouth mirror to a dentist's left hand with her right hand. All instruments are passed with their working ends pointing in the direction of use. The dentist simply keeps his or her hands in the operating position and the instruments are presented so that they are immediately ready for use (Fig. 4.7(b)).

(a)

(b)

(c)

(d)

It is often necessary for the dental nurse to exchange one hand instrument for another. She picks up the new instrument from the tray with the thumb and first two fingers of her left hand. She rotates her hand anticlockwise so that the instrument is resting between the thumb and first two fingers with her palm uppermost. The instrument is now brought in parallel with the instrument that the dentist is using (Fig. 4.7(c)). Next she takes away the old instrument with the little finger of her left hand (Fig. 4.7(d)) and at the same time places the new instrument into the dentist's hand.

It is important that instruments are exchanged in front of the patient in the 'instrument transfer zone'. This is an area around the sides and to the front of the patient's face (Fig. 4.7(b)). *Instruments should never be passed over the patient's face, and in particular not over the eyes.*

Fig. 4.7 (a) The dental nurse is picking up a mirror and probe. Note that she grasps the non-working ends.
(b) The mirror and probe are placed firmly into the dentist's hands. They are immediately ready for use.
(c) To exchange an instrument the dental nurse brings in the new instrument (a Briault probe in this picture) parallel with the instrument that the dentist is using.
(d) Exchange is completed by the dental nurse taking away the old instrument with the little finger of her left hand while placing the new instrument into the dentist's hand.

MOISTURE CONTROL

Reasons for moisture control

Fluids need to be removed from the mouth for the patient's comfort and to improve the dentist's vision. Large amounts of water from handpieces and the three-in-one syringe accumulate in the mouth, and in addition salivary flow is stimulated by dental treatment. Saliva is teeming with micro-organisms and it is preferable to exclude this extraneous infection from all cavities. In addition, salivary contamination must be avoided in certain techniques, for example pulp capping and root canal treatment.

Contamination by moisture has a detrimental effect on all filling materials and it is essential that cavities are kept dry to produce a good restoration. In this respect saliva is not the only possible contaminating fluid; crevicular exudate and bleeding from gingival margins must also be considered.

Techniques for moisture control

Aspiration

The role of the dental nurse in aspiration and cavity washing and drying has already been discussed. Since dental students will frequently have to work alone, a few comments on aspiration of water without the help of a dental nurse are relevant. Fluids can be evacuated from the mouth with a *saliva ejector*, which may be held by the patient. This is connected to a curved endpiece (Fig. 4.8). There are several designs to this endpiece, some of which incorporate a flange to retract and protect the tongue and the floor of the mouth. This is particularly valuable for the clinician working alone.

It is very difficult for the dentist working alone to see clearly when using an airotor in the upper arch since the water spray continually obscures the mirror although a little detergent on the mirror helps. Attempts can be made to move the mirror away from the spray, and the temptation to bend and work by direct vision should be resisted as far as possible.

Fig. 4.8 Two endpieces for a saliva ejector. The design on the left is made of plastic and is disposable. The metal saliva ejector on the right has a flange to retract and protect the tongue and the floor of the mouth.

Cotton-wool rolls and cellulose pads

Cotton-wool rolls are used to absorb saliva and other fluids. They are not sufficient to deal with the large volume of airotor spray but are used when restorations are being placed. They are placed in the upper buccal sulcus close to the orifice of the parotid duct (Fig. 4.9), in the lingual sulcus close to the orifices of the submandibular and sublingual ducts, and in the lower buccal sulcus. Alternatively, triangular cellulose pads can be used in the buccal sulcus.

Rubber dam

The method which gives the most complete control over moisture in the mouth is the rubber dam. The tooth or teeth to be treated, together with adjacent teeth, are placed through holes in a rubber sheet, leaving the crowns of the teeth on one side and the mouth with its moisture and infection on the other (Fig. 4.10).

The advantages of rubber dam are as follows:

Fig. 4.9 A cotton-wool roll and saliva ejector in place so that the dentist can keep the upper left quadrant dry. The retractor is being used to hold back the lip so that the cotton-wool roll shows in this photograph.

- Complete isolation of the teeth from saliva, blood, or gingival fluid exudate is possible. This is important with all restorations but particularly so in 'adhesive' restorations.

- Rubber dam aids isolation from bacteria in saliva and so is indicated when infection from the rest of the mouth must be excluded, for example in direct and indirect pulp capping and root canal treatment.

Fig. 4.10 A rubber dam in position.

- Rubber dam protects the patient from swallowing or inhaling instruments. Dentine pins, fractured burs, pieces of amalgam, wedges, crowns, inlays, root canal instruments, flanges from saliva ejectors, and even handpiece heads have all found their way into the trachea or oesophagus.

- Rubber dam protects the dentist from infection from the patient. Its use is indicated in all patients whose blood and saliva may potentially transmit disease to the dentist or his/her staff (e.g. carriers of hepatitis B).

- Rubber dam has the effect of psychologically, as well as physically, separating the dentist from the patient. Not only are water, air spray, dust, debris, and the high velocity sucker on the dentist's side of the rubber, but patients will frequently remark, with some surprise, that they feel safer with the rubber in position, or that they feel detached from what is going on, almost as if the dentist were not working on them. It is not unusual for a patient to fall asleep with a rubber dam in place.

- Once the rubber dam is in place, operative dentistry is quicker and more efficient. Wet mouths, writhing tongues, contracting lips, and garrulous patients disappear behind the rubber dam.

However, the technique has its disadvantages:

- The patient can no longer speak easily. Conversations thus become one-sided and cease.

- A few patients dislike the rubber dam intensely, feeling claustrophobic when it is in position.

- The rubber is held on posterior teeth with clamps, and a tooth which has been clamped may be sensitive for some hours after the clamp has been removed.

- The rubber dam takes time to apply and remove, although the more experienced the dentist in its use, the less time is taken. Once the rubber is in position, however, operating conditions are improved and therefore time is saved.

Rubber dam equipment
This is shown in Fig. 4.11 and consists of the following items:

Fig. 4.11 Rubber dam equipment.

Fig. 4.12 Two holes have been punched in the rubber. The one on the right hand side has not been cleanly cut and is likely to tear when the rubber is stretched.

1. Rubber dam. Rubber dam is supplied in ready-cut 15 cm (6 inches) square sheets. The rubber is resistant to tearing and it grips the teeth well and retracts gingival tissue. A dark colour (green, blue, or black) is preferred because it contrasts well with the teeth, and fragments torn off and left behind are easily seen and removed.

2. Rubber dam punch. The punch must give a clean cut otherwise there will be a weak point at the edge of the hole from which a tear may arise (Fig. 4.12). Some punches have holes of varying diameters: the larger the hole, the easier it is to stretch over a tooth; the smaller the hole, the tighter the grip.

3. Rubber dam stamp for marking the positions of the holes. This inked rubber stamp produces a series of dots on the rubber corresponding to the average positions of the teeth. When the dam is in position it should reach up to a point just below the patient's nose, thus covering the mouth but not the nose (Fig. 4.10). To achieve this when applying the rubber to the maxillary teeth or mandibular third molars, the position of the upper central incisors should be stamped about 2.5 cm (1 inch) from the top edge of the rubber sheet. For mandibular teeth the holes should be placed further up the sheet so that the rubber does not cover the nose.

4. Rubber dam clamps. These are metal clips which fit the neck of the tooth and hold the rubber dam in position. In addition, they may occasionally help to provide gingival retraction. The following clamps make a good basic set (Fig. 4.13):

Fig. 4.13 A set of rubber dam clamps. BW, JW wingless molar clamps. K, winged molar clamp. GW, premolar clamp. EW, clamp for small tooth. AW, wingless molar clamp, retentive design. Ferrier, cervical clamp, Ferrier pattern.

- BW, JW molar clamps, wingless; used when the clamp is positioned on the tooth before the rubber.

- K molar clamp, winged; the wings allow the clamp and rubber to be placed simultaneously.

- GW premolar clamp.

- EW clamp used on any small tooth.

- AW molar clamp, wingless; used on partially erupted teeth only. The jaws of this clamp are retentive and point gingivally, thus aiding retention on a tooth whose maximum bulbosity is subgingival.

- Cervical clamp, Ferrier pattern, for use on anterior teeth where retraction of rubber or gingivae is required to allow access to a cervical cavity.

5. Rubber dam clamp forceps. An instrument for placing, adjusting, and removing clamps.
6. Rubber dam lubricant. A water-based gel is supplied for this purpose but brushless shaving cream is equally suitable. A little lubricant should be applied around the holes in the rubber before sliding it over the teeth.
7. Waxed dental floss or tape. This can be used to carry the rubber past a tight contact point (see Fig. 4.17).
8. Rubber dam holder or frame. This holds the free edges of the rubber and prevents them from falling into the mouth or back against the patient's face. Several designs are available and one device is shown in Fig. 4.10.

Examples of rubber dam applications

Rubber dam application for occlusal restorations in molar and premolar teeth

Only the tooth to be treated needs to be isolated, although access is improved if more teeth are included. Since a rubber dam clamp will be required, and these can be uncomfortable, local or topical analgesia may be used even if the operative procedure itself does not require it. A clamp of suitable size is selected and tried on the tooth, placing it just coronal to the gingival margin. Floss should be attached to the holes of the clamp so that it can be retrieved should the clamp fracture across the bow (Fig. 4.14(a)).

If the dentist prefers to position the clamp before applying the rubber, a wingless clamp is selected. Having placed the clamp on the tooth, the floss is threaded through the punched and lubricated hole in the rubber dam (Fig. 4.14(b)) and the dental nurse gently pulls on the floss as the dentist slides the rubber over the bow of the clamp, first one side and then the other (Fig. 4.14(c)).

(a)

(b)

(c)

Fig. 4.14 (a) A wingless clamp in position on the upper second molar. Floss has been attached to the clamp so that the dentist can retrieve it should the clamp fracture across the bow.
(b) The floss is now threaded through the punched and lubricated hole in the rubber dam.
(c) The dentist now slides the rubber over the bow of the clamp, first one side and then the other. The dental nurse gently pulls on the floss as the rubber is placed.

(a)

(b)

(c)

Fig. 4.15 (a) A winged rubber dam clamp engaged in the lubricated hole in the rubber.
(b) Clamp and rubber are being placed on the tooth simultateously. The dental nurse should gently retract the rubber so that the dentist can see the tooth clearly.
(c) A flat plastic instrument is used to disengage the rubber from the wings of the clamp.

When it is preferred to apply clamp and rubber simultaneously, a winged clamp is chosen and the wings engaged in the lubricated hole (Fig. 4.15(a)). The dental nurse should gently retract the rubber so that the dentist can see the tooth clearly (Fig. 4.15(b)). A disadvantage of this method is that the gingival margin cannot be seen while the clamp is being placed. Once the clamp is in position, a flat plastic instrument is used to disengage the rubber from the wings of the clamp (Fig. 4.15(c)).

A piece of absorbent soft material, such as paper towel in which a hole has been cut, is now placed between the rubber and the patient's face to prevent the uncomfortable feeling of rubber against the face (Fig. 4.10). Finally, the frame is positioned.

Rubber dam application for proximal cavities in posterior teeth
The dentist must first decide which teeth are to be isolated. The more teeth that are passed through the rubber, the better will be the access. If a molar, premolar, or distal surface of a canine is to be restored, the major part of that quadrant is usually isolated; a clamp retains the rubber on the most distal tooth and a contact point holds the rubber anteriorly. Dental floss is passed through the contact points to discover what difficulties may be experienced when applying the rubber. If dental floss cannot be passed or tears, the rubber will not pass or will tear unless the cavity is partly prepared or the restoration smoothed.

Once the clamp and rubber have been placed on the most posterior tooth the rubber should be 'knifed' through each contact area (Fig. 4.16), sawing it from side to side while pressing its leading edge apically to carry it through the contact point. When a tight contact is encountered, the dentist should not spend too long on it but move to the next tooth. Once most of the teeth are through the rubber, the paper towel and the frame are applied. This improves access to deal with any remaining difficult contacts. With these the rubber should be positioned so that a leading edge of the hole is just over the contact area (Fig. 4.17). The dental nurse should hold the rubber in this position while the dentist passes floss through the contact, carrying the rubber with it. Once the floss has passed the contact it should be removed buccally and the procedure repeated until all the rubber has also passed the contact.

Finally, wooden wedges should be inserted interproximally if a bur is to be used in this area, as wedges help to reduce the risk of tearing the rubber or injuring the gingivae (Fig. 4.18).

When a matrix band has to be placed on a clamped tooth, the clamp may prevent the band from seating and therefore must be removed before the band is positioned. The band then performs the function of the clamp.

Fig. 4.16

Fig. 4.17

Fig. 4.18

Fig. 4.16   The rubber is 'knifed' through the contact area.

Fig. 4.17   The dentist flosses the rubber down through the contact point.

Fig. 4.18   A wedge is inserted to reduce the possibility of tearing the rubber or injuring the gingivae during cavity preparation.

Fig. 4.19   A strip of rubber has been placed between the upper canine and premolar to hold the rubber dam in position.

Rubber dam application for anterior teeth
Clamps are used less often in this situation. A sufficient number of teeth should protrude through the rubber for its stability and for good access. Instead of using clamps, the dam can be stabilized on the most posterior teeth to be isolated (often the canines or premolar teeth) in one of three ways:

- If there is a tight contact between the canine and premolar teeth, this will hold the rubber in position.

- The retention of rubber dam in a contact area may be improved by passing an extra strip of rubber dam through the contact (Fig. 4.19).

- Floss ligatures may be used to hold the rubber in position. Waxed dental floss is placed around the tooth and, while pulling on the ends of the floss from the buccal side, the lingual floss is pushed firmly apical to the maximum bulbosity of the tooth using a flat plastic instrument (Fig. 4.20). Finally, the floss is tied tightly in a surgical knot on the buccal side (i.e. a double throw on the first bight). It is important that the rubber is not stretched too tightly when the frame is applied since this may both restrict access and pull the rubber away from the teeth, allowing leakage.

Fig. 4.20 A floss ligature is being placed around the upper canine to hold the rubber dam in position. A flat plastic instrument is used to push the floss on the palatal side of the tooth apical to the maximum bulbosity while the floss is pulled firmly from the buccal side.

Several problems can arise when trying to apply rubber dam for cervical cavity preparations. Where a cervical cavity is to be prepared, the hole in the rubber should be placed either further buccally or lingually to the adjacent teeth, as dictated by the position of the cavity.

Retraction of the rubber is often required, and the cervical clamp should be used. To aid stability, composition may be placed over the clamp (Fig. 4.21). If the jaws of the manufacturer's clamp are not in the optimum position the clamp may be modified by heating it in a Bunsen burner flame and bending the labial jaw apically and the lingual jaw coronally.

While the cervical clamp will provide a small amount of gingival retraction, grossly subgingival caries should be uncovered by periodontal surgery at least three weeks before definitive cavity preparation. This produces a supragingival cavity with good access, and better plaque removal is possible.

Fig. 4.21 A cervical clamp has been used to isolate an abrasion-erosion cavity in the upper canine. Composition has been placed over the clamp to aid stability.

Removing the rubber dam

Once the restoration is completed the dental nurse washes and aspirates any debris from the area, and then the dentist retracts the dam buccally and cuts it interdentally with scissors. The anaesthetized lip should be protected with a finger (Fig. 4.22). Finally, the clamp, rubber dam frame, and paper towel are removed.

MAGNIFICATION

Rubber dam aids visibility and magnification improves it still further. Older dentists often find, with a decline in focusing adaptability of the eye and general visual deterioration that magnification is essential. However, it is helpful in more delicate procedures at any age, and dental students should try to gain some experience of magnification to see how much it helps them. Several different magnification systems are available varying in price by several orders of magnitude. The simpler, less expensive systems are effective and, with experience, simple to use. The more expensive, sophisticated magnifiers are less cumbersome and should have a greater depth of focus and width of field. The higher the magnification, the narrower the field of view and the greater the effect of tremor. A magnification of 2.5 times is satisfactory for most purposes, but exceptionally, 4-times magnification is used.

Fig. 4.22 When removing the dam the rubber is pulled buccally and cut interdentally with scissors. Note the dentist's finger protecting the anaesthetized lip.

Good visual discrimination in dental procedures requires good depth perception which in turn requires good binocular function. If you have difficulty with this, with or without prescription spectacles, you should ask your optician for a STREROPSIS test for binocular function. A selection of different types of magnifier (sometimes called loupes) is shown in Fig. 4.23.

Fig. 4.23 *A selection of magnifiers.*
The two on the left are the least expensive and attached to the user's own spectacles. The examples are clipped on to the dentist's prescription spectacles, but they can also be attached to safety spectacles. The magnifiers in the middle are held by a head loop, and these were popular at one time, although they are less popular now that dentists routinely wear safety spectacles to which similar, lighter magnifiers can be attached. The two magnifiers on the right are more expensive. The upper one is adjustable and so, because it can be produced in larger numbers, it is not so expensive as the lower one but is relatively heavy and the spectacles need to be held in place by a cord round the back of the head. The magnifiers at the bottom right are made specifically for the dentist with the correct inter-pupil distance, and with both the magnifiers and the surrounding lens made with the dentist's prescription built into them. The magnifiers are cemented through the main lens so that they are closer to the eye and this gives a better width of field and depth to focus. However they are very expensive.

Try to read the print in Fig. 4.24. If you have difficulty reading the text above line A, with spectacles if you wear them, then you should have your eyes tested. If you have difficulty with the text between lines A & B, magnification will help. Most dentists would need magnification to read the text below line B. The lowest line of text is 0.075 mm high (75 microns) and this compares with a stainless steel matrix band which is 50 microns thick. The printed lines are from 50 to 15 microns thick. When making inlays and crowns, the aim is to achieve a cement line at the margin of less than 20 microns.

Fig. 4.24 An eye test. Acknowledgement: This Figure has been produced with the assistance of Dr John Butler.

This typeface is used throughout this book. It is Photina and the lower case letters are 1.5 mm high (9 point)

This typeface is Univers Medium (a non-serif, i.e. unembellished font) which may be easier to read at this size—1 mm high (5 point)

This font is the smallest which is usually used in opticians' reading tests. It is 0.66 mm high (4.5 point)

A _____

Magnification may help with this 0.5 mm high font

And with this 0.33mm high font

And even more so with this 0.25 mm high font

B _____

This abnormally small type font is 0.16 mm (166 microns) high font, unreadable without magnification

These lines are:
50 microns thick   ———————
25 microns thick   ———————
20 microns thick   ———————
15 microns thick

PROTECTION, SAFETY, AND MANAGEMENT OF MINOR EMERGENCIES

There are inevitable risks in all operations and dentistry is no exception. The dentist works in the limited space of the mouth, a cavity covered by soft and mobile tissues, and at the origins of the respiratory and alimentary tracts. Sharp hand instruments, high-speed rotary instruments, and the manipulation of small objects in awkward positions provide opportunities for possible injury and mishap. However, care and forethought will greatly reduce these inherent risks.

Eye protection

An important example of such forethought is the use of plastic eye-protection spectacles for supine patients who are not already wearing their own spectacles. Eyes are vulnerable to dropped instruments and materials. These accidents should never happen because nothing should ever be passed over the patient's face. However, an inexperienced dentist or dental nurse might momentarily forget the correct position of the instrument transfer zone, and cutting debris or calculus can fly out of the mouth.

Dentists and dental nurses should also wear protective spectacles, even if their vision is normal. This is particularly important, for both dentist and dental nurse, when cast metal or amalgam is being cut in the mouth.

Airway protection

Another major consideration with a supine patient is preventing the inhalation of small objects, such as metal restorations, pins, and small hand-held files used for cleaning root canals.

Complete protection against this type of accident is provided by a rubber dam, and for this reason its use is highly desirable for many procedures, in particular root canal treatment. It may be necessary to restore a tooth before root canal treatment to allow a rubber dam to be placed. If the use of rubber dam is impossible, then files and other endodontic instruments must be secured by means of a clip and chain (a 'parachute') or by tying dental floss to them and wrapping the other end of the floss around the operator's fingers.

When fitting a restoration, such as an inlay or crown, which may also be dropped, rubber dam is not appropriate because occlusion must be checked and the rubber dam precludes this. In this case a damp butterfly sponge or a gauze square may be placed in the mouth to protect the airway while the restoration is fitted.

If a small object, such as an inlay, is lost in the mouth, the first action is to lean the patient forward and ask him or her to rinse and cough. Then the fauces and the sublingual and vestibular sulci should be examined thoroughly in that order. The tongue and palate should not be disturbed too much, because the object may be retained in the oropharynx for a short time before ingestion.

Then the patient should be got out of the chair, as far as possible without remaining in the upright position for too long, bent sharply at the hips and given one or two firm slaps on the back to help dislodge the object from the oropharynx. If a high-volume aspirator is in use the possibility of the object's having been sucked up must be checked. If all this fails to recover the object, the possibility of inhalation or ingestion must be considered. Sometimes the patient knows that he or she felt 'something going backwards' and may even know that he or she has swallowed it. However, the patient may be completely unaware of anything untoward. Quite large objects, such as a full molar crown, can fall straight through the glottis into the bifurcation of the trachea without the patient being aware of it.

Fig. 4.25 Radiograph showing a gold crown in the stomach. (Reproduced by courtesy of Professor A. H. R. Rowe.)

The next step is a thoracic radiograph to localize the foreign body in the oesophagus or stomach (Fig. 4.25) or, more seriously, in a bronchus. In the latter case, reference to an accident and emergency department or a thoracic surgeon is required because bronchoscopy and early removal is necessary to avoid pulmonary collapse.

Most objects of dental origin inadvertently swallowed can be relied upon to pass through the alimentary tract without incident. Exceptions are sharp objects such as endodontic files, which may become lodged and require surgical removal. Progress should be monitored by abdominal radiographs if necessary, and by faecal examination using a sieve under running water.

Soft tissue protection

Obviously, skilful operating is of primary importance. The insertion of sharp instruments to the correct point of application and their withdrawal without touching lips, cheek, or tongue is a basic requirement. The use of finger or thumb rests at all times and insistence upon sharp instruments are essential to good practice; blunt instruments require more force and are likely to slip. A trivial injury to soft tissue may upset a patient to an extent out of all proportion to its severity, undermining his or her confidence in the dentist.

Rotary instruments are another potential source of trauma to soft tissues. The tongue, lips, and cheeks should be retracted gently but firmly with mirrors, flanged saliva ejectors, or the flattened end of the aspirator tip, taking care to avoid pressure on the alveolar mucosa or excessive retraction of labial and buccal fraena. Rubber dam is a reliable way of retracting soft tissue. Cuts on the mucosa, should they occur, may need one or more fine sutures to bring their margins together and speed healing.

High-speed instruments are a source of risk, especially if they are bent or rotating eccentrically. The rules are as follows:

- The shank must be firmly held in the chuck, incapable of working loose.

- Bent instruments must be discarded immediately.

- Never attempt to restraighten a bent instrument because this leads to sudden fracture and a high-speed projectile is produced.

- Long tapered diamond instruments are particularly prone to bending and therefore should be examined before use. This is best done by holding the handpiece away from the patient and giving a short tap on the foot control so that the concentricity of the tip can be checked visually.

Occasionally the head of a tungsten carbide bur breaks at the neck while cutting. It should be recovered to prevent the patient swallowing or inhaling it.

Soft tissues may also be injured by careless use of caustic agents, such as the acid used to etch enamel, or hot instruments which are used occasionally to remove excess gutta-percha root canal points for example. These injuries may pass unnoticed until the local anaesthetic has worn off.

When operating on the lower teeth, inferior dental or mental anaesthesia may leave the lower lip numb for some time after the patient has left the surgery. Patients should be warned to avoid biting the anaesthetized lower lip. Some dentists leave a cotton-wool roll in the buccal sulcus to reduce the risk.

Avoiding surgical emphysema

When using an airotor or a three-in-one syringe near a breach in the mucosa or the orifice of an empty root canal, surgical emphysema may be caused by the compressed air. This is important because of the possible spread of infection into deeper tissue planes. The risk can be minimized by avoiding directing jets of air into these areas.

Dealing with accidents and accident reporting

The aphorism that 'prevention is better than cure' is nowhere more true than in the field of accident and misadventure. However, accidents will happen occasionally and there are some rules that should be followed:

- A student should inform the teacher.

- Provide whatever immediate treatment is needed (for example, sutures) or arrange other investigations such as a thoracic radiograph.

- Show the patient by your attitude and sympathy that you care for his or her welfare.

- Explain what has happened but do not be defensive or offer financial compensation.

- Make a careful record of the incident, at the time, in the patient's notes. The dental nurse should be asked to record the event as well. Retain any evidence such as broken burs.

- If the accident is serious, a qualified dentist should inform his or her protection organization. A telephone call to the dental secretary of the appropriate society is an immediate source of sound advice.

- Continue to follow up the incident carefully until it is clear that all is well.

Protection from infection

It is very important that patients and staff are protected from infection. Infection can potentially be transmitted from the dental personnel to the patient or vice versa, or from patient to patient (cross-infection). All instruments must be cleaned and sterilized (see below) between patients. Work surfaces should be disinfected by meticulous cleaning with a solution of 70 per cent isopropyl alcohol. If there is visible blood or pus, the surface should be cleaned with a disposable cloth and disinfected with hypochlorite solution containing 1 per cent available chlorine or, if the surface is metal, with 2 per cent glutaraldehyde. The solution should be left for a minimum of three minutes and the surface rinsed and dried. The surgery must be kept spotlessly clean, and regular and efficient handwashing is important. The routine use of operating gloves for all dentists and close-support dental nurses is now recommended. Cuts or abrasions should always be covered with waterproof dressings, despite the fact that gloves are worn.

The members of the dental team should take care to wash their hands meticulously before touching the patient, and hands should be rewashed during treatment if necessary.

Transmission of infection from the patient to the dental team is always important, and this is of particular relevance if the patient is known to be a carrier of a virus that may be transmitted in blood or saliva, especially hepatitis B virus, and human immunodeficiency virus (HIV). A specific code of practice is laid down for the management of known carriers of such viruses. However, since many carriers of viruses are unaware of their carrier state, only meticulous attention to sterility and cleanliness will protect the dental team. Particular care should be taken to avoid

Fig. 4.26   A needleguard to prevent needlestick injuries.

needlestick injuries, especially when local anaesthetic needles are resheathed (Fig. 4.26).

Vaccination gives safe and effective protection against hepatitis B and is becoming mandatory for all dental staff and students.

Cleanliness and sterilization of instruments

Three levels of cleanliness and sterility are used in the dental surgery:

- clean

- sterilized

- sterile at the time of use.

Many general items in the surgery should be clean but need not be sterile, for example, the hand mirror that the patient uses to look at his/her face and teeth, the washbasin taps, the handle by which the operating light is adjusted, and disposable paper tissues. Some of these, e.g. the operating light handle, should be wiped between every patient with a disinfectant but cannot be sterilized conveniently. A routine which is being used increasingly is to cover operating light handles, three-in-one syringe holders, and chair control buttons with cling film or aluminium foil which is changed between each patient.

All the instruments which enter the patient's mouth should have been sterilized. Those which penetrate soft tissues, such as needles, scalpels, and endodontic instruments, must be sterile at the time of use. Others, such as mouth mirrors, must be sterilized between patients, but it is a common and acceptable practice to store such instruments, after sterilization, in clean but not sterile drawers in the surgery.

With the increase in interest in cross-infection which has come about partly as a result of HIV, there is an increase in the use of sterile tray systems so that more instruments are sterile at the time of use.

Sterility is achieved in one of two ways:

- Using disposable sterile instruments such as needles and scalpel blades. These are mostly sterilized by gamma radiation by the manufacturer.

- Sterilizing in the surgery by means of an autoclave. Most instruments, including handpieces and three-in-one syringe nozzles, can now be sterilized in the autoclave. Instruments should be cleaned and scrubbed before being sterilized. Because of the risk of needlestick injury this should be done wearing thick rubber gloves, or preferably in an ultrasonic cleaning bath.

Disposal of waste

Sharp items, including needles and scalpels, and local anaesthetic cartridges should be placed in a rigid 'safe' container. Great care should be taken to avoid needlestick injuries to cleaners and others removing waste. Other clinical waste, which includes anything which may have been contaminated by blood (for example, cotton-wool rolls), should be sealed into stout plastic bags and kept separate from ordinary domestic waste. Local civic or health authorities have special arrangments for the disposal of clinical waste from dental practices and hospitals. The convention is to use yellow plastic bags for clinical waste which will be incinerated and black bags for non-clinical waste which is disposed of with domestic waste.

FURTHER READING

Martin, M. V. (1991). *Infection control in the dental environment*. Martin Dunitz, London.
Paul, E. (1980). *A manual of four handed dentistry*. Quintessence, Chicago, IL.

5 Instruments and handpieces

INSTRUMENTS are used to examine, clean, cut, and restore teeth. The main types are either *hand-held* or *rotary instruments* driven in a handpiece. Falling somewhere between these and the larger items of equipment dealt with in Chapter 4 are a group of auxilliary instruments which are used in operative dentistry and which will be described briefly in this chapter. These include fibre-optic lights for illumination, lights used for polymerization of certain materials, and ultrasonic scalers.

HAND INSTRUMENTS

These may be divided into instruments used for the following purposes:

- examining the mouth and teeth
- scaling
- cutting teeth and removing caries
- placing and condensing restorative materials
- carving and finishing restorations
- miscellaneous.

Instruments used for examining the mouth and teeth

Mouth mirrors

These vary in size, and although flat mirrors are most commonly used and preferred for most procedures, concave (magnifying) mirrors are also available. However, the two main types are rear-surface and front-surface reflecting mirrors (Fig. 5.1). The former has the reflective surface beneath the glass so that the image is actually seen through the thickness of the glass twice. This can produce a double image when it is necessary to look at the mirror from an angle, but the glass surface means that it is resistant to damage. Front-surface mirrors produce a clearer image, particularly at angles, and for this reason have become much more widely used in recent years. However, they are easily scratched and so care should be taken particularly during cleaning and sterilization. It is perhaps worth having both types in a standard examination kit, with the rear-surface mirror being used for general purposes and for retracting the tongue and cheeks, reserving the front-surface mirror for detailed examination.

Probes

A large variety of probes have been suggested, but many of these were designed to enable the operator to probe enamel surfaces with some vigour in diagnosing

Fig. 5.1 The two types of mouth mirror: left, front-surface reflecting; right, rear-surface reflecting. Note the double image in the rear-surface reflecting mirror.

whether or not they were carious. For reasons described in Chapter 1 this is now known to be undesirable, and a basic set of three probes is all that is usually needed (Fig. 5.2). The straight probe (actually bent, but called straight in contrast to the many curved varieties) is used for a number of purposes including checking the margins of restorations and examining caries in dentine during cavity preparation; for most of these purposes it is helpful if it is sharp. The Briault probe is another sharp probe; the design improves access to the enamel-dentine junction during cavity preparation. Many operators use this probe for the detection of subgingival calculus. The periodontal probe is blunt or has a small ball at the end; it is marked with graduations to measure the depth of periodontal pockets. These marks are also useful for a number of other measuring purposes, such as measuring the width of a tooth when a temporary crown is to be fitted. Two other types of periodontal probe are also shown in Fig. 5.2.

Fig. 5.2 Probes. From the left: straight, Briault, graduated periodontal, furcation, and CPITN periodontal probe.

Scalers

A selection of scalers is shown in Fig. 5.3. These are used for removing supra- and subgingival calculus and other deposits from teeth. They are also useful for removing temporary crowns. A periodontal textbook should be consulted for more details of the types and uses of scalers.

Instruments used for cutting teeth and removing caries

Excavators

These are used for removing softened dentine and temporary fillings. The back of the blade can also be used for placing linings, and they are sometimes used for carving amalgam. They have a discoid or ovoid blade, the margin of which is bevelled to a sharp cutting edge (Fig. 5.4).

Chisels, hatchets, and hoes

Straight and angled chisels are used for splitting off unsupported enamel. Perhaps the most useful chisel is the gingival margin trimmer (Fig. 5.5), which is a double-ended instrument with curved blades and a sloping cutting edge. It is used to trim the margins of small cavities adjacent to other teeth where access for rotary instruments is limited.

Hatchets and hoes are similar to chisels in having a straight bevelled cutting edge, and their purpose is similar. In design they are always angled or contra-angled. They differ from one another in that the cutting edge of the hatchet is in the plane of the shank (like an axe), whereas the cutting edge of the hoe lies in an axis at right angles to this plane (as in the gardener's hoe) (Fig. 5.5).

Instruments used for placing and condensing restorative materials

Plastic instruments

Some of these have flat blades and are used for conveying and shaping materials which do not involve the use of particularly heavy pressure. Some have rounded ends and are used for pushing the materials into cavities and for shaping and burnishing them. For some materials (e.g. wax) it is necessary to heat the instrument, and it is wise to set aside two or three plastic instruments which can be

Fig. 5.3 A selection of scalers. Note the angulation of the head and the extent to which some of the cutting blades are offset from the long axis of the handle.

Fig. 5.4 A selection of excavators.

Fig. 5.5 A selection of straight and angled chisels. From the left: straight, hatchet, hoe, and a pair of gingival margin trimmers for trimming mesial and distal boxes in posterior teeth.

(a)

(b)

Fig. 5.6 (a) A set of four titanium nitride instruments used for placing and shaping composite. The surface of the instrument is very hard and is not scratched by the composite filler particles. It also resists the composite sticking to it. From the left: flat-plastic, carving instrument, burnisher, plugger.
(b) Stainless steel 'plastic' instruments. From the left: amalgam condenser, burnisher, carving instrument (a half Hollenbach), flat-plastic.

heated, as regular heating tends to spoil the surface and damages the temper of the metal.

Flat plastic instruments for general use are made of stainless steel, but composite restorative materials are best placed and shaped by thin Teflon-coated or titanium nitride instruments to which the composite does not stick (Fig. 5.6(a)).

Some manufacturers produce instruments with colour-coded handles for ease of identification.

Condensers or pluggers

These are used for compressing and forming filling materials, particularly amalgam. They are used with heavy pressure. A variety of shapes and sizes are available to suit different circumstances and the end may be smooth or indented. Smooth versions are preferred as the indented type becomes clogged with old amalgam (Fig. 5.6(b)).

Carving and finishing instruments

These have sharp or semi-sharp blades of various shapes and are used to carve materials by cutting or scraping. Their smoothness is important, and so is the correct degree of sharpness. Instruments used for carving amalgam should be kept separate from those for carving wax as the latter will need to be heated and thus eventually become damaged.

HAND INSTRUMENT DESIGN

Most hand instruments are made of stainless steel or, in the case of some cutting instruments, carbon steel. Some chisels and scalers have tungsten carbide tips brazed to the cutting edge, and these retain their sharpness for much longer.

The majority of hand instruments have three parts (Fig. 5.7): the blade, the shank, and the handle. To be effective the working surface of the instrument (e.g. a chisel or scaler) must meet the surface at an angle. In some instances this angle is critical; in others it may vary over a wide range. There are many areas in the oral cavity where direct access is impossible with a straight instrument and so instruments commonly have one, two, or three bends in their shank to facilitate access to awkward places. Sometimes these angles bring the working end of the instrument back into line with the shank; sometimes it is offset (see Fig. 5.7). In general, instruments with the working tip in line with the handle are the most stable and easiest to use, but access is improved by offsetting the working tip.

The design of the handle is related to the purpose of the instrument. Instruments used primarily for tactile and exploratory purposes, for example probes, have small-diameter, light-weight handles. Instruments designed to transmit heavier pressure and which will be held for long periods of time, for example scalers, have larger-diameter, heavier handles.

USING HAND INSTRUMENTS

A hand instrument may be grasped in one of two ways:

• The *pen grip* (Fig. 5.8(a) and 5.9(a)) is self-descriptive and is most frequently used. It allows a light or a heavy touch and finely controlled movements over a wide range. The middle and ring fingers are used for support.

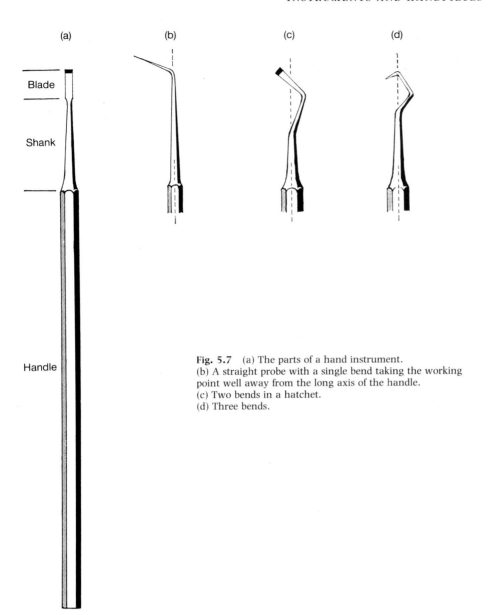

(a)   (b)   (c)   (d)

Blade

Shank

Handle

Fig. 5.7 (a) The parts of a hand instrument.
(b) A straight probe with a single bend taking the working
point well away from the long axis of the handle.
(c) Two bends in a hatchet.
(d) Three bends.

- In the *palm grip* (Fig. 5.8(b) and 5.9(b)) the instrument is held between the thumb
  and forefinger, and the handle lies across the palm and is clasped by the remaining
  fingers. The thumb is used for support. This grip, which used when operating
  upon maxillary teeth, provides heavy force over a limited range of movements but
  with greater control than with the pen grip. The *finger grip* (Fig. 5.8(c) and 5.9(c))
  is a modification of the palm grip. It is of limited value and is used when the palm
  grip fails to give the correct line of access.

The requirements of accuracy in fine movements, and of safety in forceful
manipulation, demand that *all instrumentation be accompanied by finger or thumb
support* upon adjacent firm structures, of which the firmest are the crowns of the
adjacent healthy teeth. The thumb and the third or fourth fingers of the hand
holding the instrument are the rests most often used. This is a rule which must be
closely observed; there are very few exceptions (Fig. 5.9).

Fig. 5.8 (a) Pen grip.

(b) Palm grip.

(c) Finger grip.

Fig. 5.9 (a) Pen grip.

(b) Palm grip.

(c) Finger grip.

MAINTAINING HAND INSTRUMENTS

Sharpening hand instruments

Instruments intended to cut will only do so if they are sharp. One of the main differences between an amateur and professional carpenter is the skill with which he/she identifies when his/her instruments need sharpening and how he/she keeps them sharp. All dentists should be professionals.

Steel instruments with bevelled edges, such as chisels, can be sharpened on a small flat sharpening stone (Fig. 5.10(a)) or on a mounted stone in a handpiece (Fig. 5.10(b)). Light machine oil is used as a lubricant and the instrument is held to produce a 30°–45° bevel. A fine edge initially cuts better but rapidly becomes blunt.

An alternative method (Fig. 5.10(c)), ideal for probes but also suitable for excavators and scalers, is to use a fine abrasive disc. Light pressure is used with no lubricant. Overheating must be avoided carefully. This method removes metal rapidly and gives a coarser finish to the edge, but has the advantage of speed.

Tungsten-carbide-tipped instruments retain their sharpness for very much longer than steel instruments, but when they do become blunt they are best returned to the manufacturer for sharpening.

Sterilizing hand instruments

Stainless steel, tungsten carbide, and Teflon-coated instruments can be autoclaved. Carbon steel instruments will corrode if autoclaved and then left in a wet condition. The ideal is to autoclave them in a post-vacuum autoclave which leaves the contents dry at the end of its cycle, but these are not generally available in dental surgeries.

(a)

(b)

(c)

ROTARY INSTRUMENTS

Rotary instruments, consisting of burs, stones, and discs, are small instruments held in a handpiece. The instrument is rotated in the handpiece by power from an external source, either compressed air or more directly by an electric motor. There are two broad types of equipment used to provide the rotary power covering two speed ranges:

- the airotor
- low-speed handpieces.

The airotor

The airotor (or air turbine) (Fig. 5.11) gives the highest speeds but with rather less torque than low-speed handpieces (see later). Speeds are in the range 250 000–500 000 rev/minute. These very high speeds are achieved by a small air-driven rotor or turbine mounted in bearings in the head of a contra-angle handpiece. The shank of the bur is inserted into the rotor of the handpiece and revolves with it. The handpiece always contains a system which directs water spray at the cutting head of the bur and often also contains a fibre-optic light (Fig. 5.11).

Low-speed handpieces

Low-speed handpieces are either contra-angle or straight (Fig. 5.12). The contra-angle handpiece is used almost exclusively in the mouth, and the straight handpiece is used for trimming temporary crowns or for carrying out other similar procedures outside the mouth. The speed of these handpieces is less than that of the airotor but the torque is greater. Most handpieces are equipped with a water spray for use in the higher speed ranges. The speed ranges are given in the caption to Fig. 5.12, and although the handpieces are called 'low-speed' to distinguish them from the airotor, which will only operate at very high speeds, some of them operate at speeds approaching that of the airotor.

The drive for low-speed handpieces comes from a small electric motor attached directly to the handpiece, and the speed of this is controlled by a foot control or a control on the electric motor or on the dental unit. An alternative, which is usually less expensive, is an air motor, again attached directly to the end of the handpiece. Low-speed handpieces can be rotated clockwise or anti-clockwise, whereas the airotor only rotates clockwise.

Fig. 5.10 (a) Sharpening a chisel on a flat oil stone.
(b) Sharpening an excavator with a mounted stone in a straight handpiece.
(c) Sharpening a chisel with a disc in a straight handpiece.

Fig. 5.11 Airotor handpiece in operation showing the waterspray and also the fibre-optic light system.

Fig. 5.12 A selection of low-speed handpieces. From the left.
1:1 ratio contra-angle handpiece used for most procedures. Latch-grip burs are used. Commonly identified with a blue coloured band on the shank of the handpiece and a blue dot on the head. Speed in the range 4000–40 000 rev/minute.
1:4 ratio speed increasing handpiece. Takes friction grip burs and operates in the speed range 16 000–160 000 rev/min. Commonly identified with a red band. Useful for finishing cavity preparations and also finishing restorations.
7:1 ratio speed reducing handpiece. Takes latch-grip burs and is used for drilling pin holes and other procedures where a slow speed is indicated. Operates in the speed range 550–5500 rev/min and is commonly identified with green bands.
A straight handpiece which takes straight burs or may be modified to take latch-grip burs. A 1:1 ratio handpiece is identified with a blue band and reducing speed is identified with a green band. Used to trim temporary restorations and other similar procedures. Usually used outside the mouth.

Maintaining and sterilizing handpieces

Modern handpieces are autoclavable and should be autoclaved between patients. Most handpieces should be lubricated before and after autoclaving using a lubricant delivered from an aerosol can through an adaptor (Fig. 5.13) or by an air-driven cleaning and lubricating machine (Fig. 5.14).

Fig. 5.13 An aerosol lubricant being used with a low-speed handpiece. Different adaptors for the nozzle of the aerosol are available for each type of handpiece. The paper towel is used to absorb excess lubricant coming through the head of the handpiece.

Fig. 5.14 An automatic handpiece cleaning unit which is connected to the air supply. The shield at the front is rotated out of the way and the handpiece plugged onto the connector. A detergent is then flushed through the handpiece followed by oil, both of which come from refillable containers at the back of the unit. This is a more efficient and quicker system than using aerosols.

Burs and stones

A selection of burs and stones is shown in Figs 5.15, 5.16, and 5.17.
Rotary cutting instruments are retained in the handpiece by one of three methods:

- friction—in the older type of airotor
- a latch grip—in the contra-angle low-speed handpiece

Fig. 5.15 A selection of friction grip burs for the airotor. From the left: three tungsten carbide burs, three diamond burs, and three special metal cutting burs (Beaver) which have gold-coloured shanks to help identify them. Note the very fine cross-cuts on the cutting blades.

Fig. 5.16 A selection of steel latch burs for use at low speed. From the left: three round burs of different sizes, three straight cross-cut fissure burs, a tapered cross-cut fissure bur, and an inverted cone bur.

Fig. 5.17 Similar sizes of steel and tungsten carbide burs. The head of the tungsten carbide bur (right) can be seen attached to a steel shank. The head is a slightly different shape.

- a quick-release clamping chuck—in the straight handpiece and now in most contra-angle, low-speed handpieces, and airotors.

The cutting end of the instrument consists of either a set of blades of tungsten carbide or steel, or abrasive material, ranging in hardness from diamond to sand, embedded in a suitable medium.

Airotor burs

Burs used in the airotor always have friction grip shanks and the cutting end is diamond or tungsten carbide. These hard materials are necessary because of the very high speeds (Fig. 5.15).

Airotor burs are used to cut sound enamel and dentine and to remove existing restorations. They should not be used to remove caries because they cut too fast and the sense of 'feel' is lost (see p. 101). When cutting enamel some operators prefer diamond and some tungsten carbide burs. However, ceramic materials are best cut with diamond burs while all other restorations are best cut with tungsten carbide. Special tungsten carbide burs (Beaver burs) are produced to cut metal restorations in the mouth. Diamond instruments cut cast metal very slowly and ordinary tungsten carbide burs tend to break.

A very large selection of shapes of burs is available and advice will be given in later chapters on the choice of bur for specific procedures.

Low-speed burs

As with airotor burs a large selection of shapes is available (Fig. 5.16) which include:

- round burs

- flat fissure burs which are parallel-sided and have blades which may be plain or cross-cut to increase efficiency

- tapered fissure burs which may also be plain or cross-cut

- inverted cone burs.

All these burs are available in a range of sizes which are numbered according to the diameter of the cutting tip.

Steel, diamond, and tungsten carbide low-speed burs are available. Steel burs are not expensive but have a short working life because they are rapidly blunted by enamel and will rust after autoclaving if they are not dried. Tungsten carbide burs run more smoothly than steel and they can be autoclaved; therefore they are becoming more popular than steel. Many dentists now discard steel burs after a single use (Fig. 5.17).

Round burs are used to remove soft carious dentine at slow speed. The steel bur will not cut sound dentine or enamel very quickly at low speed, and so the experienced clinician can feel his/her way around a cavity, removing softened dentine and leaving sound dentine behind. Round burs are used because, as caries spreads out in dentine simultaneously in all directions, carious lesions in dentine are often naturally round.

Stones

These are made of abrasives such as carborundum (green) or alundum (white or pink) which are moulded into a range of shapes and fixed directly to a bur shank (Fig. 5.18). They can be used in the final stages of tooth preparation for smoothing the surface, but are more commonly used for shaping, smoothing, and finishing cast metal and porcelain restorations out of the mouth. For this purpose they are usually used at medium speeds in the straight handpiece.

Fig. 5.18 A selection of stones mounted on latch-grip shanks and three straight-shank instruments. The instrument on the far right is a diamond-coated instrument for use in the laboratory or at the chairside for coarse adjustment of restorations and appliances.

Finishing instruments

Burs and points

In addition to burs for basic cavity preparation, a whole range are produced for finishing preparations and restorations. These are made of steel (for amalgam) or of very fine diamond particles or multifluted tungsten carbide (for composite) (Figs. 5.19 and 5.20).

Discs

Rigid and flexible discs are available with abrasive materials of different degrees of coarseness applied to one surface (or occasionally both). Some discs also cut at their edge. All discs are used mounted on mandrels which are usually of a screw design, although some flexible discs are designed to be used with snap-on mandrels so that they can be changed easily. Rigid discs are used in a straight handpiece outside the mouth for cutting and trimming such things as posts and temporary crowns. They are no longer used in tooth preparation because of the risks of injury to the patient

Fig. 5.19 Finishing instruments for amalgam. From the left: five plain-cut plain steel finishing burs, two mounted stones, three mounted abrasive rubber points from coarse to fine, and a mounted abrasive rubber cup.

Fig. 5.20 Composite finishing instruments. Across the top is a plastic finishing strip with a blank area in the middle to facilitate passage between the teeth. On the right the abrasive is coarse and on the left it is fine. From the left: a mounted fine white stone, two medium grit composite finishing diamonds, two fine grit composite finishing diamonds, a mounted abrasive rubber disc, a mandrel for the two abrasive single-sided flexible discs which are snap-fit onto the mandrel, and four colour-coded flexible abrasive discs mounted on plastic stubs which fit the mandrel to the right of the picture.

even with the use of a disc guard. Flexible single-sided discs are commonly used for finishing composite and other restorations, and are available in a wide range of grits and sizes (Fig. 5.20).

Abrasive strips

Hand-held flexible strips of metal, plastic, or linen with abrasive on one side can be used to finish restorations. Metal strips are sometimes used to remove overhanging amalgam ledges on old restorations, but they are not very effective and are traumatic to the gingival papilla (see Chapter 11). Plastic strips are used to finish composite restorations on the approximal surfaces of teeth (Fig. 5.20).

Maintaining and sterilizing burs and stones

All burs and stones should be autoclaved, although if steel burs are re-used they should be dried quickly after autoclaving otherwise they will corrode. Flexible discs and strips are disposable.

Tungsten carbide burs become blunt and diamond burs become clogged or the diamond particles become lost or worn. They should be assessed regularly and discarded when they have completed their useful life. Tungsten carbide burs occasionally break in use and diamond burs become bent. A bent bur should always be discarded immediately.

Tooth preparation with rotary instruments

Speed, torque, and 'feel'

The speed ranges used in tooth preparation are shown in the caption to Fig. 5.12. Torque is the *turning moment* of the instrument. In a high-torque cutting system, considerable pressure can be applied to the surface being cut by means of the bur with only minimal slowing of the drive, although other factors such as heat, vibration, and the amount of material removed may rise conspicuously. Broadly speaking, the higher is the speed the lower is the torque. It is more efficient to cut hard materials such as enamel, porcelain, and metal at high speeds and to cut softer materials such as carious dentine at lower speeds with higher torque.

An important characteristic of cutting systems is the 'feel' which the operator senses through the handpiece. At high speed there is very little 'feel' and the cutting must be controlled visually. This is difficult because of the water spray. At lower speeds 'feel' is useful in controlling the cutting process, particularly close to the pulp. This is the principal reason why low-speed sharp burs should be used for removing carious dentine.

Heat generation and dissipation

Heat is generated in proportion to the work done and is potentially damaging to a vital pulp. High-speed cutting always produces sufficient heat to necessitate a cooling water spray, and in most airotor systems the water spray comes on automatically when the foot control is depressed. Prolonged slow-speed cutting also generates heat, and most low-speed handpieces now have a built-in water spray although this may have to be switched on when it is required. In the finishing stages of preparation too much water spray can hinder vision, and at that stage very little tooth tissue is being removed and hence little heat is being produced. Therefore it is usual for the water spray not to be used and for the dental nurse to wash and dry the cavity at frequent intervals, which serves the dual purposes of improving visibility and cooling the tooth.

One of the many advantages of using natural extracted teeth in preclinical practical courses is that occasionally an inexperienced student will cut enamel and dentine without sufficient cooling and the distinctive burning smell pervades the classroom. This is a good lesson because, once recognized, the students know that they must *never* produce this smell in clinical work.

Effects on the patient

Tooth preparation with rotary instruments has the potential of producing pain, vibration, pressure, trauma, and long-term effects on the pulp.

Provided that cooling is adequate (and the water is not too cold), superficial preparation of the enamel is not painful. However, cutting dentine in a vital tooth is painful and local analgesia is usually used. High-speed cutting of enamel produces intense localized heat, even with apparently effective cooling. As an illustration, the reader should try cutting an extracted tooth with the airotor in a darkened room with eyes dark-adapted.

The range of perceptible vibration is limited and rotary instrumentation at speeds over 40 000 rev/minute produces high-frequency vibrations above the normal range of perception. Therefore patients usually prefer the airotor to tooth preparation at lower speeds.

An electric motor drive may produce less vibration than an air motor, particularly when the air motor, which has more moving parts, becomes worn. Therefore electric motors are preferred, although they are more expensive and the maintenance costs are usually higher.

Another source of vibration is the attachment of the bur to the handpiece. Friction grip shanks have no movement between the bur shank and the chuck, whereas conventional latch burs are a looser fit and therefore are capable of vibration. An increasing number of handpiece systems now have friction chucks which grip latch bur shanks more firmly and produce less vibration. The chuck is released by a button at the back of the handpiece head.

Very little pressure is used in cutting at high speed, as pressure would slow the bur and reduce cutting speed. Greater pressure is used at lower speeds and higher torques, and this must be carefully controlled or the patient will find it uncomfortable.

Sharp revolving instruments used at awkward angles in the restricted confines of a mouth which moves independently of the operator give rise to real risks of accidental damage. This is a principal reason why the undergraduate student must develop a high level of skill in the use of the full range of rotary instruments before starting clinical work. Even experienced dentists occasionally cause damage to tissues around the tooth. Accidental and unexpected exposure of the pulp (a traumatic exposure) sometimes results from careless cutting or from variations in, or a lack of understanding of, pulpal anatomy. Proper examination of the pre-operative radiographs, and care, should avoid these injuries. Damage to sound adjacent teeth in the preparation of approximal surfaces is commonplace and difficult to avoid. Usually the damage is minor and may not be seen. However, it does create plaque-retentive areas on the adjacent surface and increases the risk of development of a new carious lesion. Great care should be taken to avoid these injuries by using appropriately sized and shaped burs, and hand instrumentation when appropriate. Good illumination is essential and magnification helps. The adjacent teeth are sometimes physically protected with a matrix band (see Chapter 7).

It is not always possible to avoid some injury to the gingival margin adjacent to the cavity being prepared. Proper selection of bur shapes and sizes and the use of rubber dam or gingival retraction with cord (see Chapter 10) will help, but in any case such minor injuries usually heal with no long-term ill effect.

It is difficult to disentangle the effects of caries, tooth preparation, and the restorative materials when pulp changes occur. All dentists will find that teeth which they have restored occasionally suffer acute or chronic pulpitis or degenerative or necrotic changes in the pulp. If this occurs frequently, it is because the dentist is being too optimistic about pulp prognosis, or is being traumatic in tooth preparation, or there is something wrong with the restorative materials or techniques being used. One of the things that should be checked is that water cooling is sufficient.

Choosing the bur for the job

Skilled and experienced clinicians often use a limited number of burs from the very wide variety produced for the same purpose and obtain equally satisfactory results. However, the inexperienced student needs to start somewhere, and it is better for the clinical teacher to suggest a range of burs than for this to be prescribed in a textbook. However, clinicians will experiment with new designs of bur throughout their practising lifetimes, and it is an important part of postgraduate continuing education to read catalogues, visit dental trade exhibitions, and generally seek better ways of making preparations.

The illustrations in Chapters 6–10 show a number of burs being used for specific purposes, and in some cases these are designed especially for that purpose. There is a saying 'a bad workman blames his tools', but the corollary is that a good workman knows which tool does the job best for him/her.

Surface finish

For most purposes a relatively smooth finished enamel surface is preferable, although the faster cutting systems generally produce rough surfaces. Therefore many preparations consist of two stages, the initial rapid tooth reduction followed by more precise shaping and finishing. As a general rule straight-cut burs provide a smoother finish than cross-cut designs and tungsten carbide burs provide a smoother finish than either steel or diamond burs.

Finishing and polishing restorations

The surfaces produced by various finishing instruments on composite are shown in Fig. 5.21. The margins and surfaces of restorations should be smoothed and polished so that plaque retention is minimized. There is a wide and increasing range of instruments to do this, in particular instruments for finishing composite materials. Ideally, any material should be shaped properly in its unset stage so that it requires minimal finishing with medium or fine abrasive instruments. If more shaping is necessary, a coarser instrument should be used first. Several finishing systems—for example disc systems—have four grades of abrasives. It is not always necessary to start with the coarsest, but one of the finest should be used at the end of the procedure.

(a)

(b)

Fig. 5.21 The surface of composite (a) as left by a matrix strip and (b) finished with a coarse abrasive disc. Field width for both, 30 μm. (Reproduced by courtesey of Dr M. O. Atta.)

AUXILIARY INSTRUMENTS AND EQUIPMENT

Very good illumination for cavity preparation can be obtained with fibre-optic lighting systems producing illumination at the head of the handpiece (Fig. 5.22). These are available in both airotor and low-speed handpieces. Independent fibre-optic lighting has also been used as well as, or instead of, the normal operating light, and fibre-optics have been built into some mouth mirrors.

Many restorative materials are now polymerized by the application of intense visible light. The light is transmitted from its source down a flexible light guide which is either a fibre-optic cable or a gel. The end of this is applied to the tooth.

Fig. 5.22 A fibre-optic lighting system built into the head of a contra-angle low-speed handpiece.

Fig. 5.23 Two types of curing light, one with a flexible light guide and the other as a hand-held instrument with a rigid light guide. An eye-protection shield is also shown.

Alternatively, the light can be contained in a hand-held piece of equipment connected to the electrical supply. In this case the short light guide is rigid and more robust (Fig. 5.23). Rechargeable versions, which are simply left parked in the charging unit while not in use, are now available.

All systems produce light of such intensity that it can be damaging to the retina and so it must not be shone in the direction of the patient's, operator's, or dental nurse's eyes, and so protective screens or spectacles are used. One of these is shown in use in Fig. 8.9(h) (p. 146).

Many surgeries are now equipped with ultrasonic and electrosurgical equipment. Ultrasonic scalers are a quick and efficient way of removing calculus. The working tip is vibrated at ultrasonic frequency under voluminous water spray. Their use is described fully in textbooks of periodontology. Ultrasonic instruments are also used with special files in endodontics (see textbooks on endodontics) and have other uses such as loosening crowns or posts when they have to be removed (see textbooks on crowns and bridges). Electrosurgical equipment, with a fine point or loop electrode, is occasionally used, for example to remove hyperplastic gingival tissue, to gain access to cavity margins, or to expose the margin of a tooth fractured below gingival level.

6 Treatment of pit and fissure caries

INTRODUCTION

Occlusal, buccal, and cingulum pits and fissures are obvious stagnation areas where plaque can form and mature, anatomically protected from even a single toothbrush filament by the dimensions of the fissure. Clinical studies continue to show a high and unremitting attack on permanent molars in children despite the overall reduced prevalence of caries in many areas of the developed world. The concept of dental caries being exclusively a disease of young newly erupted teeth is not tenable. Clinical studies of children aged between 10 and 16 years have shown that occlusal surfaces that had been erupted for seven to ten years were still developing clinical lesions.

Early diagnosis is difficult since the early enamel lesion may form out of sight around the walls of the fissure (Fig. 1.12). The prerequisites for diagnosis are sharp eyes, magnification, dry clean teeth, a probe to remove plaque from the fissure (but not to be forced into it), and good bite-wing radiographs (see p. 10).

The operative management of occlusal caries varies according to the state of health or disease of the fissure system. A fissure system judged as clinically and radiographically caries-free can be protected by a *fissure sealant*. This is a layer of resin or glass ionomer cement applied to enamel which has been treated so that the restorative material adheres to the tooth surface.

Alternatively, where caries is obvious in part of the fissure system, either clinically or radiographically, it is removed and the cavity can then be lined and restored with a composite resin whilst a fissure sealant is used to protect the remaining fissure system. This is a *sealant restoration* (or a *preventive resin restoration*).

Another possibility is to restore the missing tooth tissue with *amalgam*. In this case, consideration must be given to the remaining fissure system to decide whether it should be included in the cavity preparation so that adjacent areas, judged as likely to become carious, are also restored. These operative alternatives will now be considered in greater detail.

FISSURE SEALING

Indications

Sealing of susceptible pits and fissures is carried out as soon after eruption as possible. First, second, and third permanent molars are obvious candidates, but all molars are not automatically fissure sealed. However, caries or missing teeth which have been extracted because of caries in a child's mouth indicates caries risk and will favour the use of sealants. Similarly, if a young adult requires restoration of one second molar, fissure sealing the remaining second molars seems to be a logical preventive measure. Fissure morphology is also relevant. A fissure pattern of shallow rounded grooves is unlikely to decay, but a deep fissure pattern is more susceptible since it is difficult to clean. Where the dentist believes that the patient's diet contains frequent sugar intakes or when poor oral hygiene cannot be improved—for example with handicapped patients—fissures should be sealed.

Finally, the tooth to be fissure sealed must be capable of being isolated from salivary contamination since contamination while placing the sealant is the most common cause of failure. At best, salivary contamination will result in the sealant falling off, with no permanent harm. At worst, however, the sealant will be partly retained but leak, so that caries can progress beneath it, safe from salivary protection, fluoride ions, and detection by the dentist. Therefore good isolation from saliva is an essential part of the clinical technique, with a rubber dam being the preferred method.

Clinical technique for resin sealers

Anaesthesia and isolation

If necessary a little local anaesthetic is infiltrated or topical anaesthetic is applied to avoid discomfort from the rubber dam clamp.

Cleaning

The tooth surface to be etched and sealed may be cleaned with a bristle brush in a handpiece and a pumice and water slurry. Oil-based polishing pastes or those containing fluoride should not be used, as these may interfere with etching. The pumice is washed away using the three-in-one syringe and a sharp probe is dragged through the fissure system. This will remove some of the deeper plaque that the brush cannot reach. In this case it does not matter if there is some damage to partly demineralized enamel in the neck of the fissure because the fissure is to be sealed. The tooth is then washed again and dried thoroughly.

Etching

The tooth is now etched with phosphoric acid (30–50 per cent) (see Chapter 3). The acid etchant is supplied by the manufacturer in the form of either a colourless liquid or a coloured gel. The etchant is applied over the whole occlusal surface extending onto the lingual or buccal surface where grooves require sealing (Fig. 6.1(a)). Etching the entire occlusal surface avoids the danger of covering an unetched surface with sealant and thus inviting leakage. The acid can be applied with a tiny pledget of cotton wool, a sponge, or a brush. Alternatively, the gel can be placed accurately with a disposable syringe and blunt needle. As soon as the complete area to be etched is covered with acid, the time is noted and the enamel is etched for 30 seconds. When acid is used in the liquid form, fresh solution can be dabbed on the surfaces during etching, but care should be taken to treat the enamel surface very carefully and not rub the cotton-wool pellet or sponge on the surface during acid application as this may damage the fragile enamel lattice-work being formed.

Washing

After 30 seconds the acid is washed away. Initially a water jet from the three-in-one syringe is used to remove most of the acid. If a rubber dam is not in place, careful aspiration is important to avoid damage to soft tissue by the acid. After approximately 5 seconds of water, the air button is also pressed, forming a strong water-air spray which should be played over the etched surface for 20–30 seconds. With coloured gels, it is tempting to stop washing when the colour has gone.

(a) (b) (c)

(d) (e)

Fig. 6.1 (a) A brush is used to apply the etchant gel over the occlusal surface of the tooth to be fissure sealed.
(b) Dried etched enamel appears matt, white, and frosty.
(c) The sealant is applied to the etched surface using a small disposable brush or a syringe with a disposable tip.
(d) Light curing a fissure sealant.
(e) A fluoride-containing varnish is applied to the etched enamel at the periphery of the restoration where it has not been covered with sealant.

However, the purpose is not just to remove the surplus acid, but to flush the precipitates out of the newly formed etch pits, and this takes a full 20–30 seconds.

Drying

It is good practice to check that the airline is not contaminated by water or oil by blowing it at a clean glass or paper surface. The tooth surface is now thoroughly dried with air from the three-in-one syringe. This drying is most important since any moisture on the etched surface will stop penetration of the resin into the enamel. A minimum of 15 seconds drying is recommended. At this stage the etched area should appear matt, white, and frosty (Fig. 6.1(b)). With rubber dam, there should be no danger of salivary contamination of the etched surface. If this does occur, however, it is essential to re-etch the enamel because adherent organic material in saliva will block the pores and it cannot be removed completely even by vigorous washing.

Applying the sealant

Fissure sealants are supplied both as light-curing and chemically curing materials. A light-cured resin does not require mixing but a chemically cured resin has two components which are gently mixed together with a brush.

The sealant is applied to the etched surface using a small disposable brush or applicator supplied by the manufacturer. The sealant is applied to the etched pits and fissures and up the etched cuspal slopes (Fig. 6.1(c)). If a light-cured material has been chosen, the light should be placed directly over the sealant but should not touch it (Fig. 6.1(d)). With a molar tooth, if the light source is of a smaller diameter than the tooth it should be directed at the distal part of the occlusal surface for the full curing time recommended by the manufacturer of the resin and then moved mesially for a similar period. Any buccal or palatal groove or pit should be similarly cured with the light source directly over it. Since the polymerizing lights are potentially damaging to the operator's eyes, special eye-protective glasses should be used or the dental nurse should hold a special filter screen in the operator's line of vision (see Fig. 8.9(h)). Some lights have protective cups which can be placed over the end of the light guide.

Most chemically cured sealants polymerize in 1–3 minutes and the manufacturer's instructions should be followed.

The outer surface layer of any sealant will not polymerize, due to the inhibiting effect of oxygen in the atmosphere. The sealant will therefore always appear to have a greasy film after polymerization. Finally, a fluoride-containing varnish is applied to the etched enamel at the periphery of the restoration where it has not been covered with sealant (Fig. 6.1(e)).

Checking the occlusion

The rubber dam is now removed and the occlusion checked with articulating paper. Whilst it is considered acceptable to allow any high spots to be abraded away when unfilled resin fissure sealants are used, with the lightly filled materials it is wiser to reduce high spots by grinding with a small round diamond stone in a low-speed handpiece.

Clinical technique for glass ionomer cement sealers

A glass ionomer cement should only be chosen for fissure sealing when the fissure is wide enough for entry by a probe. Where fissures are not patent, either a very small tapered diamond bur (Intensiv D2) should be used to open them prior to fissure sealing or a resin sealant should be chosen. The advantage of the glass ionomer material is that it contains fluoride and therefore is cariostatic. However, these materials have not yet been investigated as fully in clinical trials as the resin sealants (Fig. 6.2).

The tooth to be sealed is isolated and the fissure is cleaned with ten per cent polyacrylic acid conditioning agent supplied by the manufacturer for 30–60 seconds. It is then washed and dried, and the glass ionomer material, mixed to a consistency which will still just flow, is applied along the fissure and firmly burnished into position. Excess material is easily removed with the burnisher. A layer of unfilled BIS GMA resin (enamel bonding resin used with composite) is applied to the glass ionomer cement and light cured to prevent it drying out while it completes its setting reaction. Finally, the occlusion is checked and should a 'high spot' require reduction a further layer of varnish is applied to protect the freshly set material.

Fig. 6.2 A glass ionomer fissure sealant which has been in place for 14 years. (Reproduced by courtesy of Dr John McLean.)

THE SEALANT RESTORATION [OR PREVENTIVE RESIN RESTORATION]

Indications

The sealant restoration was born out of the use of pit and fissure sealants. It is a natural extension of the technique where pit and fissure decay is minimal or in cases where the operator is unsure whether there is decay present. It allows such dubious areas to be investigated by cutting with a very small bur, and it is also useful in situations where caries has progressed into dentine yet is still confined to a rather small part of the fissure system. The technique restores the carious area and seals the rest of the fissures.

Clinical technique

Cavity preparation

A local anaesthetic is given. Rubber dam is applied and the tooth is thoroughly cleaned as before (Fig. 6.3(a)). A small, pear-shaped tungsten carbide bur (Jet 330) or a small tapered diamond (Intensiv D2) is now used in the airotor to widen slightly and deepen the fissure and to gain access to caries. If the carious enamel is removed and no dentine caries is found, there is no need to extend the preparation.

If caries has extended into dentine, the airotor is used to remove the minimum amount of enamel necessary to gain access to caries (Fig. 6.3(b)). A small round bur is now used in the low-speed handpiece to remove carious dentine, which is often stained, from the enamel-dentine junction. During this process the access cavity may require further enlargement to allow access to caries on the enamel-dentine junction. Thus high- and low-speed handpieces are used alternately so that the cavity is kept as small as possible commensurate with removing all the caries from the enamel-dentine junction. This area should be stain-free and feel hard when a sharp probe is run along it.

When the enamel-dentine junction is caries-free, any soft caries overlying the pulp is removed with either a slowly rotating round bur in the slow-speed handpiece or a sharp excavator (Fig. 6.3(c)) (see Chapter 3).

Lining and etching

If the cavity is larger than expected, the deep dentine is covered with a calcium hydroxide-containing cement (Fig. 6.3(d)). A second layer of radiopaque glass ionomer may be placed in a deep cavity (Fig. 6.3(e)). In a shallower cavity a radiopaque glass ionomer cement may be used alone to replace the missing dentine. The polyacrylic acid conditioning liquid supplied by the manufacturer should be applied to any exposed dentine with a brush or small pledget of cotton-wool. After 10 seconds the cavity is washed and dried and the glass ionomer cement placed. Once this material has set, any glass ionomer material on the enamel walls should be removed with an air rotor. The enamel walls of the cavity and the occlusal surface of the tooth are now etched with acid (Fig. 6.3(f)). After 30 seconds this is washed and dried as before (Fig. 6.3(g)).

Filling the cavity

A universal composite resin, or one specifically designed for use in posterior teeth, is selected. It is supplied with a bonding (unfilled) resin which should be painted on the etched enamel walls and occlusal surface and blown with dry air to form a thin layer, avoiding puddles of material in the cavity. The resin is polymerized with light as before (Fig. 6.3(h)).

The cavity is now filled with the posterior composite (Fig. 6.3(i)). These light-cured materials will not cure reliably in depths exceeding 2 mm. Thus, if the cavity is deeper than this (a graduated pocket measuring probe can be used to check depth) the material must be placed in increments. Each increment is then cured before the next is placed, taking care not to dispense more than is needed because normal light in the surgery will polymerize the unused material. An increment of composite is placed or syringed directly into the cavity and gently nudged into position using a small 'non-stick' instrument. Care should be taken not to trap air under the material. When the final increment is placed an instrument is used to shape the occlusal surface, restoring cuspal inclines in the larger cavity before light curing the material. Better still, the glass ionomer material is brought up to the enamel–dentine junction to replace all the missing dentine so that only one increment of composite, the thickness of the enamel, is required (Fig 6.3(i)).

The remaining fissure system has already been covered by the unfilled bonding

Fig. 6.3 (a) A lower second molar isolated with rubber dam prior to placing a sealant restoration.
(b) Enamel is removed to gain access to obvious caries.
(c) Soft caries over the pulp is removed.
(d) Exposed dentine is covered with a calcium hydroxide-containing cement.
(e) A second layer of glass ionomer lining may be placed in a deep cavity.
(f) The enamel walls of the cavity and the occlusal surface of the tooth are etched with acid.
(g) Etched enamel after washing and drying.
(h) Bonding resin is applied to the cavity walls and occlusal surface.
(i) The cavity is filled with composite resin. Use of the glass ionomer lining in this tooth allowed the composite to be placed and cured in a single 2 mm increment.
(j) A fissure sealant is applied to the whole occlusal surface.
(k) The occlusion is checked with articulating paper which will locate areas of occlusal contact with a coloured mark.

resin. A layer of fissure sealant is now painted over the entire occlusal surface and polymerized (Fig. 6.3(j)). Alternatively, posterior composite resin can be gently agitated with a plastic instrument into the adjacent pits and fissures, and light cured to act as a heavily filled pit and fissure sealant.

Finishing the restoration

Excess resin is carefully removed with 12-bladed tungsten carbide finishing burs or with fine diamond composite finishing burs (Fig. 5.20). Once the rubber dam has been removed, the occlusal contacts should be checked with thin articulating paper (Fig. 6.3(k)). This is placed between the dried teeth and the patient is asked to move the teeth over each other as if eating. Any 'high' spot on the restoration will be located by a mark and can be reduced; the aim is to have the restoration in harmonious occlusion. The restoration can finally be smoothed with alumina-impregnated rubber points.

LARGER POSTERIOR COMPOSITES

It is not uncommon for occlusal caries to undermine the occlusal enamel widely (Figs 6.4(a) and 6.4(b)). In the past such restorations have often been restored with

(g)

(h)

(i)

(a)

(b)

(c)

(d)

(e)

(f)

Fig. 6.4 (a) A large occlusal cavity is present in the lower first molar.
(b) Access to caries begins to reveal the extent of the lesion.
(c) The enamel–dentine junction is made caries-free, soft caries is excavated over the pulp, and a calcium hydroxide-containing cement is placed in the depth of the cavity.
(d) Much of the missing dentine is replaced by a second lining of glass ionomer cement. Today this would be brought up to the enamel–dentine junction and only one increment of composite would be required.
(e) An increment of composite being light cured.
(f) The final increment of composite can now be placed.
(g) The completed restoration.
(h) The restoration after five years.
(i) The restoration after nine years. There is some wear, but the margins are intact and the restoration can still be considered a success. If this wear was thought to be excessive, the surface layer of composite could be removed and the restoration resurfaced with more composite. Such repairs, or maintenance procedures, are not possible with amalgam. Modern composites are likely to be more durable than the materials available when the restoration was placed.

amalgam after all the overhanging enamel has been cut away. With posterior composite materials and glass ionomer cements, it is now possible to use these adhesive materials to restore the missing tooth tissue and support the remaining enamel without needing to remove so much of it.

Therefore once caries has been removed decisions have to be made about the strength of the remaining tooth tissue. Figure 6.4(c) shows a large occlusal cavity with a considerable amount of overhanging enamel. This cavity was restored with a calcium hydroxide lining over the deepest part of the cavity followed by a layer of glass ionomer cement to replace much of the missing dentine (Fig. 6.4(d)). Finally, the enamel walls were acid etched and the remainder of the tooth restored with a posterior composite which was built up in increments as described previously (Figs 6.4(e), 6.4(f), and 6.4(g)). The same restoration is shown after five and nine years in Figs. 6.4(h) and 6.4(i).

Fig. 6.5 A 25-year-old occlusal amalgam restoration. Although the restoration is somewhat pitted and ditched, it is still serviceable.

THE AMALGAM RESTORATION

Indications

While the use of composite and sealant restorations seems particularly appropriate for the management of the small carious lesion in posterior teeth, some dentists still regard amalgam as the material of choice in larger cavities where the restorative material must take considerable occlusal force (Fig. 6.5).

Clinical technique

Pre-operative procedures

Where a bite-wing radiograph shows occlusal caries into dentine, an extensive restoration can be predicted. Where caries appears to approach the pulp on a bite-wing radiograph, the vitality of the pulp should be tested and a periapical radiograph should also be taken to check the state of the periapical tissues. A tooth showing extensive dentine caries should always be tested for vitality before giving a local anaesthetic. A tooth with a necrotic pulp must be root filled before being restored, but before this is done the feasibility, type, and extent of the coronal restoration should be determined. The ultimate objective is a functional crown and if this is not possible, the tooth should be extracted.

Where extensive destruction of the occlusal surface is predicted it is useful to check the occlusion with articulating paper so that a mental note can be made of occlusal contacts. This information will be useful during cavity preparation and when carving the restoration.

If the radiograph shows extensive dentine caries, a rubber dam should be used. Perfect moisture control is important in deep cavities because micro-exposures can be present and the prognosis for pulp capping is better if the pulpal wound is not contaminated with saliva.

Access to caries and clearing the enamel-dentine junction

The enamel overlying the carious dentine is removed with a small pear-shaped tungsten carbide bur in the airotor (Jet 330) (Fig. 6.6(a)).

After access to the carious dentine has been gained, a round bur in a low-speed handpiece is used to remove all soft caries and stain from the enamel-dentine junction. During this process the access cavity may need to be enlarged to remove overhanging unsupported enamel and allow adequate vision of and access to the enamel-dentine junction. This region is judged to be caries-free when all visible stain has been removed and when it is no longer sticky to a sharp probe.

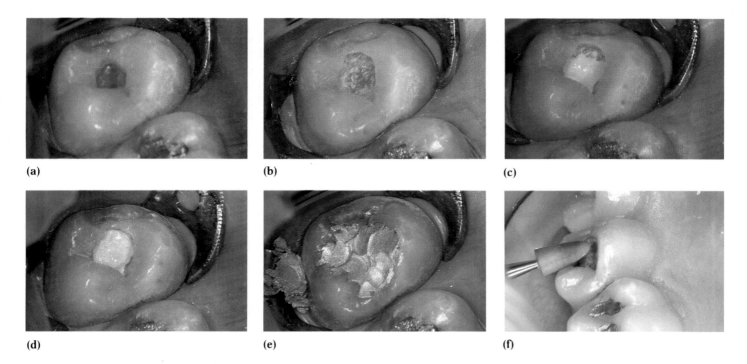

(a)

(b)

(c)

(d)

(e)

(f)

At this stage any remaining overhanging enamel should be removed with the airotor because enamel which is not supported by dentine and/or an adhesive restorative material is brittle and liable to fracture under occlusal stress. This is one of the stages in cavity preparation when examination of the occlusion before the preparation may prove useful. A mental note can be made of areas of occlusal contact where it is particularly important to avoid overhanging enamel.

Examine and treat the remaining fissures (extension for prevention)

Thus far the shape of the cavity preparation has been entirely determined by the spread of caries at the enamel-dentine junction. Now, any remaining fissure pattern must be carefully examined. If the remaining fissures are extensive, it is usually best to reconsider the decision to use amalgam and instead place a sealant restoration (see earlier). This would be indicated particularly in a young patient with a high caries rate and a deep fissure system. In an older patient, with a lower incidence of disease and a shallow fissure pattern or one obliterated by tooth wear, this would not be necessary, and a simple amalgam or composite restoration without extension would be sufficient.

Traditionally, before the current approaches to preventing caries were developed, the usual procedure was to continue the cavity preparation into the sound non-carious fissures in the hope that this would prevent caries developing in them. This 'extension for prevention' is now considered to be unnecessary destruction of sound tooth tissue and is no longer practised.

The retention of the restoration: amalgam-margin angles

Preparing the cavity in this way will result in a cavity whose widest part is determined by the spread of caries at the enamel-dentine junction. Thus, it will be retentive for amalgam (Figs. 6.7(b) and 6.7(c)). Figure 6.7(a) shows a diagram of a cavity where caries necessitated the cavity being wide at one end but narrow at the other where it extends along a fissure with minimal caries. The two lines represent the sections shown in Figs. 6.7(b) and 6.7(c). Both sections show the cavity to be undercut and thus retentive.

Fig. 6.6 (a) An amalgam restoration is to be placed in the upper second molar. The airotor is used to gain access to caries.
(b) The enamel-dentine junction is caries-free and soft caries is removed over the pulp.
(c) A calcium hydroxide-containing lining is placed over the pulpal surface.
(d) A second lining (an EBA cement) is placed and cavity varnish applied.
(e) The amalgam is overpacked prior to carving.
(f) An abrasive rubber point is used to polish the occlusal amalgam.

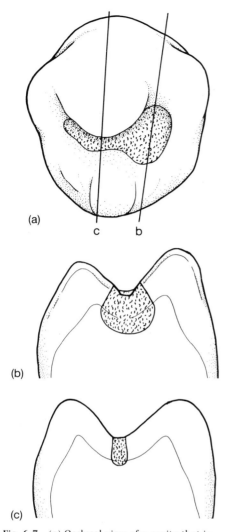

(a)

(b)

(c)

Fig. 6.7 (a) Occlusal view of a cavity that is wide at one end, reflecting the extent of the carious lesion, but as narrow as possible at the other end where it extends along a fissure with minimal caries. The two lines indicate the sections shown in Figs 6.7(b) and (c).
(b) Section through the wide part of the cavity. Note the widest region is at the enamel–dentine junction where the spread of caries would be greatest. The base of the cavity is rounded as a result of excavation of caries. The cavo-surface angles are prepared to about 100°–110° so that amalgam-margin angles of at least 70° can be achieved.
(c) Section through the narrow part of the filling after placing amalgam. The occlusion allows this to be carved flat thus achieving very high amalgam-margin angles. (By courtesy of Professor Richard Elderton and Dental Update).

Angulation of the Jet 330 bur as in Fig. 6.7(b) has resulted in a cavo-surface angle of about 105 degrees in these regions. This is important because it will allow the amalgam to be carved with an amalgam-margin angle in excess of 70 degrees without interfering with the occlusion. This has been shown to be a critical measurement with amalgam since amalgam-margin angles less than this tend to break in clinical service (see p. 180) resulting in 'ditched' margins. In Fig. 6.7(c) the cavo-surface angle is again about 105 degrees, but in this part of the filling, where there is no opposing occlusal contact, the amalgam can be carved flat, thus achieving very high amalgam-margin angles.

Removing caries over the pulp

Caries over the pulp is now removed with a sharp excavator or slowly rotating round bur. The management of deep caries in this area has already been discussed in Chapter 3. Remember that stained but hard dentine should be left over the pulp in a symptomless vital tooth and subsequently covered with a calcium hydroxide lining (Fig. 6.6(b)). This procedure, *indirect pulp capping*, kills remaining bacteria, allows the formation of reparative dentine, and allows partial remineralization of the dentine remaining in the base of the cavity.

Cleaning the cavity

The final stage of cavity preparation is to clean the cavity thoroughly with water and air spray. The cavity is then dried with air, but not overdried as this may damage the pulp.

Lining and varnishing the cavity

Where removal of carious dentine has resulted in the floor of the cavity being close to the pulp a calcium hydroxide lining is required (see p. 65) (Fig. 6.6(c)).

In a very deep cavity a second layer of lining material may be required. A glass ionomer cement is suitable for this purpose. This lining is placed so that there is sufficient room for 2–2.5 mm of amalgam over it (Fig. 6.6(d)). It is very important to be sure that no trace of lining material remains on the enamel cavity walls because eventually this would dissolve in the oral fluids, leaving a wide gap between the restoration and the tooth and inviting recurrent caries.

Finally, a cavity varnish can be applied to the cavity walls. Varnishes are natural or synthetic resins in a solvent, such as chloroform, and they have been shown to prevent initial leakage around freshly packed amalgam restorations. Eventually, it is thought, they are replaced by corrosion products of the alloy, but until this happens they resist secondary caries and protect the pulp from bacterial insult. Two layers of varnish are used, each applied with a small pledget of cotton-wool and blown dry. The resulting layer is some 3 μm thick.

Perfect moisture control is essential when amalgam is placed; thus if a rubber dam is not being used, dry cotton-wool rolls and a saliva ejector should be inserted. If an occlusal cavity has a buccal or lingual extension, a matrix band is needed to replace the missing wall (see p. 123).

Choice of amalgam

This is not a textbook of dental materials but reference to such a book is essential at this stage if the student is to understand how to handle the material. Amalgam alloys contain silver, tin, copper, and often zinc. Alloys containing a higher proportion of copper are preferred as they corrode less than the alloys used in the past and show minimal distortion of the set restoration (creep) (see p. 52).

The alloy particles are lathe-cut (irregularly shaped), spherical, or a mixture of the two. It is essential to know which of these alloys is being used because they handle

Fig. 6.8 An amalgamator with a capsule of amalgam in position behind a shield (A). The appropriate card is chosen from the rack (B) and inserted into the slot (C). The electronic control is then activated.

quite differently. Lathe-cut alloys must be firmly condensed into position; they resist packing pressure and are hard work to handle. Spherical alloys, however, can be condensed into a cavity with much less force and larger-diameter instruments may be needed to handle them.

Amalgam alloy is mixed with mercury before being packed into the cavity. The alloy and mercury are supplied in a capsule with alloy at one end and mercury at the other, separated by a diaphragm which is broken just before placing the capsule in an amalgamator (Fig. 6.8). These capsules have the advantage that the manufacturer has placed the optimal quantity of alloy and mercury in the capsules and thus a consistent mix should be assured. They also have the safety advantages that liquid mercury does not need to be stored in bulk in the surgery, reducing the risk of spillage, and as the mixing is carried out in a closed capsule there is less risk of air contamination by mercury vapour.

Alternatively, it is still possible to obtain alloy and mercury in bulk for insertion into a mechanical amalgamator. This machine volumetrically dispenses portions of alloy and mercury and mixes them together.

With all amalgams the manufacturer will recommend the mixing time and this will vary according to the alloy selected. Similarly, the working time of the particular alloy will also have been determined by the manufacturer. Therefore it is possible to select alloys with long or short working times. Dental schools usually select alloys with long working times for undergraduate use because undergraduates are bound to work slowly at first.

Inserting the amalgam

The mixed alloy is transferred to a suitable container and a small amount is picked up in an amalgam carrier and transferred to the cavity. Sometimes this procedure presents problems because gravity can help the amalgam fall straight out again! The trick is to push the amalgam carrier firmly towards the base of the cavity and keep it in this position while expelling the amalgam.

The condensing instrument of choice is a double-ended plastic instrument with a flat/smooth condensing surface (see Fig. 5.6(b)). The diameter of the tip must be such that it can be accommodated on the floor of the cavity at its narrowest point, otherwise condensation of the deepest layers of amalgam is impossible.

Condensation proceeds by pressure on the amalgam mass in the centre of the cavity and then stepping the condenser towards the walls of the cavity and the ends of the fissures. Only when the first increment has been condensed adequately, should the next increment be added. It is wrong to suppose that the earlier layers inserted can later be condensed by heavy pressure in the later stages of packing. Only porosity close to the surface would be eliminated, and voids would remain in the deeper part. In addition, there would be poor union between the increments.

As the amalgam level reaches the cavity margins, packing continues to allow an excess to build up over the ultimate level of the finished restoration (Fig. 6.6(e)).

Carving the amalgam

Amalgam should not be carved until it is sufficiently firm. The amalgam is carved with a sharp carving instrument (e.g. 1/2 Hollenbach). The carver is held so that its blade lies across the margin of the filling, half on tooth and half on amalgam, moving parallel to the margin. In this manner small increments of amalgam are removed, defining the margin of the restoration. In a narrow restoration (Fig. 6.7(c)) no attempt should be made to reproduce the natural fissure pattern, but the amalgam can be carved flat to ensure a strong amalgam margin angle. In a larger restoration, cuspal slopes should be carved and fissures may be delineated.

Great care should be taken to achieve a smooth and uniform surface whilst the mass is still capable of being carved. The occlusion should be checked by removing the rubber dam or cotton-wool rolls and asking the patient to place the teeth lightly together. If no abnormal contact is felt, the patient should be asked to grind the teeth gently as if eating. Sometimes the restoration will feel 'high' to the patient and then a brightly burnished mark will be seen on the amalgam surface, which is otherwise matt in texture. Articulating paper is useful to localize a high spot, particularly in patients who, when anaesthetized, find it difficult to say whether a restoration feels 'high'. The restoration should not be overcarved so that occlusal contacts are lost and the occlusion left unstable, allowing the tooth to over-erupt.

Finally, the restoration should be smoothed with a tightly rolled pledget of cotton-wool.

Polishing

In the past it has been considered essential to polish amalgam restorations to attain a high gloss, thus aiding plaque control and reducing corrosion. However, some studies have shown that polishing may not be essential with the new high copper content amalgam alloys. Comparison of polished and unpolished high copper content alloy restorations after a year of clinical service showed a similar surface finish.

If an amalgam restoration is to be polished, this should not be done until at least 24 hours after it has been placed. The surface should first be inspected to detect any heavily burnished spots which may indicate areas where excessive load is being exerted. Such areas should be reduced with a steel finishing bur which may also be used to run lightly over the whole area. Only the lightest pressure should be necessary, as the aim is to smooth the restoration, not remove it from occlusion. The finishing bur is followed by a series of abrasive rubber points (Fig. 6.6(f)), the shapes of which are particularly suited to polishing the fissure surfaces. As in all polishing procedures, success depends upon the use of a light uniform touch and the constant movement of the instrument over the carved surface. Care should be taken to retain the carving and avoid overheating the amalgam and thus damaging the pulp.

When the surface presents a uniform 'satin' finish, a final polish may be given with a soft cup-shaped brush or rubber cup and a fine abrasive. A proprietary dentifrice or zinc oxide powder moistened with methylated spirit is suitable.

THE CHOICE OF MATERIAL FOR RESTORATIONS OF PITS AND FISSURES

Because amalgam has been used for so long, it is still the 'default option' or automatic choice of material for many established dentists. However, with today's better understanding of the carious process and its prevention, with many lesions presenting in a less advanced state, and with recent improvements in alternative materials, the choice should now be carefully considered rather than following habit and tradition. Several relatively long-term studies now show good success rates for small composites compared with amalgam, and the modern materials are likely to perform better than the materials which were in use when these studies were performed (compare Fig. 6.4(i) and 6.5).

Composites have the advantages of being repairable and of bonding to the enamel surface. When used only as an enamel replacement material over glass ionomer which replaces all the dentine, composite is simple to place in one increment.

It is often said that the posterior composites are 'technique sensitive', i.e. flaws in technique will cause failure. This is true, but the same argument pertains to amalgam. A contaminated composite will often fail immediately, either by falling out or discolouring, whereas a saliva-contaminated amalgam will look satisfactory at first but the moisture incorporated in the amalgam will cause expansion which will show later as ditching around the margins (Fig. 11.17).

Taking these considerations into account, the current recommendations for restoring occlusal caries are shown in Fig. 6.9.

• Examine bite-wing radiographs very carefully for evidence of dentine caries.	
• Vulnerable teeth with no clinical or radiographic evidence of dentine caries	Fissure seal
• Early dentine caries, suspected clinically because of grey stain visible through apparently intact enamel (Fig. 6.3(a))	Sealant restoration
• Definite dentine caries on radiograph but with minimal breakdown of enamel	Radiopaque glass ionomer–composite layered restoration
• Larger lesion with more loss of occlusal enamel but with occlusal contacts still on enamel	Glass ionomer to replace all or most of the dentine and composite or amalgam to replace the enamel
• Large cavity where the occlusal contacts will be primarily on the restoration	Amalgam at present but keep the success of the new composite materials under review
• Replacing failed amalgams	If small, replace with a sealant restoration or a glass ionomer–composite layered restoration; if large, replace with amalgam (see Chapter 11).

Fig. 6.9 Current recommendations for restoring occlusal caries.

FURTHER READING

Elderton, R. J. (1984). Cavo-surface angles, amalgam-margin angles and occlusal cavity preparations. *Br. Dent. J.* **156**, 319–24.

Smith, B. G. N., Wright, P., and Brown, D. (1994). *Clinical handling of dental materials* (2nd edn). John Wright, Bristol.

7 Treatment of approximal caries in posterior teeth

INTRODUCTION

Stagnation areas exist on the approximal surfaces of posterior teeth, cervical to the contact areas, where plaque can form and mature. Unless an interdental cleaning agent such as dental floss is used, this plaque is difficult to remove mechanically and thus caries may develop. In its early stage this lesion is not visible clinically and so good bite-wing radiographs are essential for diagnosis (see p. 11).

The management of approximal caries varies according to the state of disease of the surface. Thus, caries confined to the enamel on a bite-wing radiograph should be encouraged to arrest. Dietary advice and showing the patient how to floss this particular approximal surface are important. Fluoride in the form of toothpaste or a mouthwash should be used, and in some cases, where patient co-operation is doubtful, chairside application of fluoride by the dentist may also be indicated. The patient should understand that the lesion must be checked again by the dentist both clinically and radiographically, usually in six months.

In contrast, once caries is visible in dentine on bite-wing radiographs, operative treatment is usually indicated, in addition to preventive measures, to restore the integrity of the tooth surface (Fig. 7.1).

Access to caries may be gained in several ways:

- occlusally, by cutting through the marginal ridge

- occlusally, leaving the marginal ridge intact

- buccally or lingually, leaving the marginal ridge intact

- direct access, which is possible if the adjacent tooth is missing.

Occlusal access through the marginal ridge is the approach that has been used most extensively over the years, with the cavity being filled with amalgam. With the development of adhesive restorative materials (composite resins and glass ionomer cements) specifically for use in posterior teeth, new techniques are being developed and tested for these materials. One innovation is the possibility of leaving the marginal ridge intact, approaching the caries occlusally, buccally, or lingually and filling the cavity with an adhesive material. This approach is only suited to relatively small lesions where caries has not undermined the marginal ridge to such an extent that it collapses during cavity preparation.

Each of these operative alternatives will now be considered in greater detail. In addition, techniques for restoring badly broken-down teeth with amalgam will be described.

Fig. 7.1 A bite-wing radiograph showing a large lesion in dentine on the distal aspect of the upper first premolar. Lesions are also obvious in dentine on the mesial and distal aspects of the lower first molar. All these lesions were managed operatively as well as preventively. In contrast, earlier lesions in the lower first premolar, distal; lower second premolar, mesial and distal; upper second premolar, mesial and distal; and upper first molar, mesial, were not treated operatively.

APPROXIMAL AMALGAM RESTORATION: ACCESS THROUGH THE MARGINAL RIDGE

Pre-operative procedures

The vitality of the tooth is checked and a local anaesthetic is given if necessary. Rubber dam is applied to the quadrant and a small wooden wedge is inserted interdentally between the carious tooth and the adjacent tooth (Fig. 7.2(a)). This prevents the rubber from being caught and torn by burs.

Access to caries and clearing the enamel–dentine junction

Access is gained to the carious dentine with a small pear-shaped tungsten carbide bur (e.g. Jet 330) in the airotor. The bur is placed centrally on the inner aspect of the marginal ridge and angled slightly towards the contact area of the tooth so that it is directed towards the area of affected dentine. The operator will feel the bur suddenly drop into the carious dentine because all resistance to penetration disappears. The cavity is widened slightly bucco-lingually to gain access to the carious dentine beneath. Note that a small sliver of enamel is left at the contact area to prevent accidental damage to the adjacent tooth (Fig. 7.2(b)). If this precaution is not taken, the risk of damaging the approximal surface of the next tooth is very high and this is a serious, if common, failure of technique. Any occlusal extension to gain access to occlusal caries is conveniently cut at this time. It is important to be conservative of tooth tissue so that the tooth remains as strong as possible and the occlusal forces placed on the amalgam are as small as possible. However, if the tooth is caries-free occlusally, it is not necessary to cut out the fissure.

The sliver of enamel in the region of the contact area can now be fractured out with a small chisel (Figs. 7.2(c) and 7.2(d)). Subsequently, a round steel bur (the size will vary according to the size of the cavity) is used in the low-speed handpiece to clear caries from the enamel-dentine junction buccally, lingually, and cervically (Fig. 7.2(e)).

Finishing the enamel margins

Any carious or unsupported enamel is now removed. Although the airotor bur can be used again approximally at this stage, a gingival margin trimmer is often ideal for the purpose. Initially, the instrument is used as a hatchet with a cutting stroke to trim the buccal and lingual aspects of the approximal part of the cavity (Fig. 7.3(a)). It is then swept round cervically (Fig. 7.3(b)) where the angulation of the blade at 25° to normal (Fig. 7.3(c)) removes unsupported enamel at the cervical margin.

The resulting outline of the approximal part of the cavity is thus determined by the extent of the caries, taking the form of a sweeping curve (Fig. 7.3). Since caries begins cervical to the contact area, removal of carious tissue and unsupported enamel will usually leave the cavity margins clear of the adjacent tooth bucally, lingually, and cervically. The resulting margins are thus accessible to instrumentation by the dentist and cleaning by the patient and will not hinder matrix band placement. They can also be checked visually for recurrent caries at subsequent appointments. The margins should not be extended buccally or lingually more than necessary. Wherever caries allows, the gingival margin should be supragingival as subgingival margins encourage plaque accumulation and therefore gingival inflammation and recurrent caries.

This cavity design is conservative of tooth tissue and should minimize damage to adjacent teeth during cavity preparation. However, where the operator is worried about cutting the next tooth, a steel matrix band may be placed around it. Unfortunately, this will not reliably prevent damage to the adjacent tooth and hinders access, which probably explains why few experienced practitioners use it.

The rounded approximal outline facilitates thorough condensation of the

(a)

(b)

(c)

(d)

(e)

(f)

(g)

(h)

(i)

(j)

(k)

(l)

(a)

(b)

(c)

amalgam in the gingival area. Using the cervical margin trimmer cervically removes friable spicules of enamel which would otherwise fracture when the matrix band is placed (Fig. 7.2(f)). Occlusal and approximal parts of the cavity should merge smoothly with each other. Further occlusal extension into the occlusal fissures is only undertaken when caries and/or an existing unsatisfactory occlusal restoration is present.

Removing caries over the pulp

Having established the outline of the cavity and finished the enamel walls, caries over the pulp is removed with a slowly rotating round bur or sharp excavator.

Retention

Since amalgam is not adhesive to enamel and dentine, the cavity must be designed to retain the filling. If the cavity has been prepared as described, it will be undercut and therefore will resist forces tending to dislodge the filling occlusally. However, there is the possibility that the filling may fracture and/or slide out of its cavity towards the adjacent tooth.

Where occlusal caries and/or removal of an old restoration have required occlusal cavity preparation, this is used to hold the approximal part of the restoration in place

Fig. 7.3 Use of a gingival margin trimmer on an extracted tooth.
(a) The instrument is initially used as a hatchet with a cutting stroke to trim the buccal and lingual aspects of the cavity.
(b) It is then swept around cervically.
(c) The angulation of the blade, at 25° to normal, removes unsupported enamel at the cervical margin.

Fig. 7.2 (*left*) (a) The cavity on the distal aspect of the upper first premolar is to be restored. The radiographic appearance of this lesion is seen in Fig. 7.1. Rubber dam is applied and a wooden wedge is inserted interdentally.
(b) A small bur is used to gain access to caries. On the distal aspect, the cavity is widened slightly bucco-lingually, and a small sliver of enamel is left at the contact area.
(c) The sliver of enamel in the contact area is fractured out with a small chisel.
(d) A round steel bur can now be used in the low-speed handpiece to clear caries from the enamel–dentine junction.
(e) The enamel–dentine junction is made caries-free. Carious undermined enamel remains on the cervical floor.
(f) The enamel walls of this cavity have been finished with a cervical margin trimmer. Note the different appearance of the cervical floor when compared with Fig. 7.2(e).
(g) The axial wall of the cavity is lined with a cement containing calcium hydroxide. The occlusal part of the cavity is just into dentine and does not require lining.
(h) A matrix retainer and a curved band are in place. Wedges are positioned buccally and palatally to ensure good cervical adaptation. The band is burnished to contact the adjacent tooth.
(i) The first stage of carving is to adjust the height of the marginal ridge by removing a fillet of amalgam from against the matrix with a sharp probe.
(j) Carving is nearly complete. The rubber dam is now removed so that the occlusion can be checked.
(k) Articulating paper is used to mark areas of occlusal contact.
(l) The completed polished restoration.

by making the occlusal part (the 'lock') dovetail-shaped (Fig. 7.2(f)). However, it is not necessary to cut away further sound tissue occlusally since the approximal part of the cavity can be made self-retentive. This is done by cutting retention grooves in the dentine of the axio-buccal and axio-lingual walls of the box (Figs. 7.4(a) and 7.4(b)). These are cut with a small round bur.

The use of a round bur to remove caries from the enamel–dentine junction gingivally will usually result in a groove in this area (Fig. 7.5). Thus the curved floor will be inclined slightly inwards and will be at right angles to the long axis of the tooth. In addition to helping to retain the filling, this shape potentially resists the forces of occlusion which would otherwise tend to force the restoration out of the cavity (the glacier effect).

Lower premolars

Caries on the approximal surfaces of lower premolar teeth can present difficulties in cavity preparation, particularly in the lower first premolar where the occlusal surface is angled lingually and the occlusal fissure is lingually placed. Where caries necessitates an occlusal extension this should, if possible, be cut at the expense of the

Fig. 7.4 (a) Retention grooves on an extracted tooth cut with a small round bur in the dentine of axiobuccal and axiolingual walls. The arrow points to the retention groove on one side of the cavity.
(b) A clinical example.
(c) The restored tooth.
(Figs. 7.4(b) and 7.4(c) reproduced by courtesey of Dr P. B. Robinson.)

(a)   **(c)**

(b)

Fig. 7.5 Diagram showing how the use of a round bur to remove caries cervically results in the floor being inclined slightly inwards (the left-hand side of the cavity). This will help to retain the filling and potentially resists the forces of occlusion which would otherwise tend to force the restoration out of the cavity. On the right-hand side of the cavity the gingival floor takes the unfavourable shape of an inclined plane sloping outwards, and so the restoration will tend to fracture. (Reproduced by courtesy of Professor Richard Elderton and Dental Update.)

Potential fracture site

Lining

Unfavourable inclination of gingival floor

Favourable inclination of gingival floor

buccal cusp, although its position will be dictated by the caries. Angulation of the bur at right angles to the occlusal surface helps to avoid undermining the small lingual cusp. In these teeth, approximal and occlusal parts of the cavity are frequently cut at different angles (Fig. 7.6).

Lining and varnishing the cavity

This procedure is similar to that described for an occlusal amalgam preparation except that the axial wall must also be lined. Care should be taken not to block out the retention grooves. The angle between the pulpal floor and the axial wall (pulpo-axial line angle) should be rounded to make the amalgam maximally strong in this area (Figs. 7.2(g) and 3.8).

Applying the matrix band

When placing amalgam in the cavity the aim is to restore the contact area and marginal ridge and at the same time have the smoothest possible junction between the restoration and the tooth. However, since the cavity is incompletely enclosed, an extra wall must be provided if amalgam is to be contained and firmly condensed. This extra wall is provided by a metal strip—a matrix band. The functions of the matrix band are as follows:

• to retain the amalgam in the cavity during condensation

• to permit the close adaptation of the amalgam to cervical and axial margins

• to help to restore the contact area and external contour of the crown.

Matrices are of three types:

• The band encircles the tooth and is secured by a retainer on the buccal or, in some cases, the lingual aspect. This is the commonest form and there are many patterns of this type of retainer. In addition, there are many different designs of band—straight, curved, and contoured (Fig. 7.7). The chief advantage of this type is that it can be firmly adapted to the tooth (Fig. 7.2(h)).

• The band encircles three-quarters of the crown and is retained by jaws impinging into the free embrasure (Fig. 7.8). It is particularly useful where contact points are so tight that it is difficult to place the other types of matrix band.

• This type includes a number of variations in which only a matrix band is used, without a retainer. The matrix strip may be wedged in position, may be retained by a ligature, or may be a complete band tightened by a spring mechanism (Fig. 7.9). It has the advantage that no retainer is needed and is particularly well suited to badly broken-down teeth (see p. 136).

The most important features of a good matrix are that the band should be thin (about 0.05 mm), smooth, and strong, it should be capable of close adaptation, in particular to the cervical margin, and finally it should allow the contact with the adjacent tooth to be restored otherwise food packing will occur. When the matrix band is placed it should be stretched in the contact area by careful burnishing (Figs. 7.2(h), 7.8 and 7.9). This is particularly important where a spherical amalgam alloy has been chosen because it is rarely possible to push the contact out during condensation with this type of alloy. The width of the band should allow it to extend 1.0 mm above the marginal ridge to allow for overpacking of the restoration, but it should not be too tall otherwise access is restricted.

The adaptation of the matrix at the cervical margin is very important. The problem is that the occlusal circumference of the tooth is greater than the cervical circumference and access to trim away any excess of amalgam in this area is poor.

Fig. 7.6 A lower premolar cavity prepared on a carious extracted tooth.

Fig. 7.7 There are many different designs of matrix band. This figure shows examples of straight, curved, and contoured bands.

Fig. 7.8 In this design of matrix retainer the band encircles three-quarters of the crown. The matrix band replaces the mesial wall of the cavity. A wedge has been inserted from the lingual side to ensure good cervical adaptation and the band is burnished to contact the adjacent tooth.

Fig. 7.9 There is no matrix retainer with this design of band. The band is tightened around the tooth by a spring mechanism.

Fig. 7.10 A Siquveland matrix retainer in use. Note the adjustment of the toggle to reduce the circumference of the band cervically. A wooden wedge has also been placed. A gap is present bucally and a second wedge would be useful. However, it is difficult to insert with this matrix retainer because the toggle is in the way.

Curved bands are designed to help solve this problem. An alternative solution is to select a design of matrix retainer which is adjustable, to allow a straight band to be pulled into a truncated cone (Fig. 7.10). As well as this it is also necessary to use a cervical wedge (usually wood) to push the band firmly against the tooth and hold it in position with sufficient force to prevent amalgam escaping between the band and the tooth under packing pressure (Figs. 7.2(h), 7.8, and 7.9).

While it should hold the band firmly in position cervically, the wedge should not be of such a height that it prevents the formation of a contact point. Thus the wedge must be triangular in cross-section, with the base of the triangle resting on the gingiva. Since the dimensions of the triangle and space to be filled will vary from tooth to tooth and from mouth to mouth, a variety of sizes of wooden wedge should be available. Another function of the wedge is to separate the teeth slightly so that when it and the matrix are finally removed, the teeth return to their original positions, closing the small space left by the thickness of the matrix band.

The matrix band is gently passed between the contact points so that its lower edges lie just over the cervical margin of the cavity. The band is then tightened and a wedge inserted. The contact area is burnished against the adjacent tooth. When the cavity is wide bucco-lingually, it may be necessary to slacken the matrix band retainer slightly to achieve this. If so, wedging is particularly important to hold the band in place, and wedges should be inserted from both buccal and lingual sides (Fig. 7.2(h)). This approach may also be useful on the mesial surface of the first upper premolar where the concavity of the canine fossa requires careful wedging.

Before inserting the amalgam, a final check should be made of the following points:

- Is the matrix system stable?

- Does it fit the cervical margin? It should not be possible to insert a probe between the cervical margin and the band. If a small space remains which cannot be eliminated because of a groove in the tooth (e.g. mesially on the upper first premolar teeth), remember where it is and remove excess amalgam in this region as soon as the matrix band is removed (Fig. 7.10).

- Has the band been burnished in the contact area so that the contact point can be restored?

- Is the height of the band sufficient?

- Is the cavity clean and dry?

Inserting the amalgam

This procedure is similar to that described for an occlusal amalgam restoration except that the first increment of amalgam is directed into the deepest approximal part of the cavity. Great care must be taken to condense the amalgam thoroughly in this critical gingival area. It is helpful to slide the packing instrument from side to side to ensure adaptation of the filling material to the axial walls. The amalgam should be overpacked as described previously.

With a spherical alloy, broader condensing instruments can be used to advantage. This favours quicker condensation and better control of the mass of amalgam. It reduces the tendency to penetrate rather than consolidate the more mobile mass which is characteristic of this type of amalgam.

Carving and finishing the amalgam

Initially, the height of the marginal ridge should be adjusted to that of the next tooth. This is done by removing a fillet of amalgam from against the matrix with a sharp probe (Fig. 7.2(i)) and then reducing the height of the ridge with a carver.

After removing the wedge, the retainer is loosened and removed. The band is first removed from the contact point not being restored. It is then wrapped back against the tooth adjoining the new restoration. From this position it can be lifted in an axial or oblique direction free of the filling; alternatively, one end of the band can be cut off short near the embrasure with scissors and the remaining end pulled through laterally to clear the contact area. Some dentists support the marginal ridge with a pledget of cotton-wool held on the amalgam condenser when removing the band.

Sometimes the marginal ridge is broken off when the matrix band is removed, destroying the occlusal form. This may happen for several reasons: poor cavity preparation, insufficient condensation of the marginal ridge, or inadequate trimming of the ridge before removing the band. It is obviously important to diagnose the cause of the problem before replacing the amalgam so that the same mistake is not repeated.

Once the band is removed, the axial and cervical margins are now accessible. The axial margins are trimmed towards the gingivae with a downward stroke of a sharp carver. The gingival margin should require only the lightest of trimming with a carver inserted into the embrasure, unless an excess has been anticipated (see p. 124).

Once the occlusal surface has been carved (Fig. 7.2(j)), the rubber dam is removed and the occlusion checked and adjusted (Fig. 7.2(k)). The patient should be asked to put his teeth together gently and, if no abnormality is noted, a light 'rubbing' movement is requested. As before, the aim is to reproduce occlusal contacts, not eliminate them. Light burnishing and smoothing completes the finish at this stage. Care is taken to see that all residual fragments of amalgam are removed from the interdental space by dislodging them with a probe and using the water and air spray from a three-in-one syringe.

The restoration may be finished after 24 hours, following much the same sequence as described for the occlusal restoration (Figs. 7.2(l) and 7.4(c)). The contact area is not polished, but the amalgam cervical to it can be smoothed with a fine abrasive strip.

APPROXIMAL COMPOSITE RESTORATIONS: ACCESS THROUGH THE MARGINAL RIDGE

Indications

Many dentists still regard amalgam as the material of choice for approximal restorations. However, it suffers the disadvantages of poor appearance, a lack of adhesion to dental tissues, and no cariostatic properties. Amalgam will obturate a hole, but it will not support enamel and dentine. For these reasons, where appearance is of particular importance, or where enamel and dentine are weakened by caries, a posterior composite resin restoration may well be indicated.

A particular problem exists when composite is used to restore approximal cavities. At the gingival floor of these cavities there is a thin layer of enamel or, if caries has progressed further, the gingival floor may be in dentine. Composite resins shrink as they set. The bond to the enamel of the axial walls will be stronger than the bond to the thin enamel or dentine cervically and so the material may shrink away from the weaker bond. In other words, a space may be created at the cervical margin. The fact that the materials are light cured actually exacerbates this phenomenon since the composite will contract towards the light source, i.e. away from the cervical margin. The larger the cavity, the greater is the potential shrinkage. The solution (as with occlusal restorations) is to fill the bulk of the cavity with glass ionomer cement, sometimes including the whole of the cervical floor, and then restore the occlusal surface with a layer of composite. The alternative is to pack the composite in increments, curing each in turn before placing the next.

Any adhesive material is very susceptible to moisture contamination while being placed. For this reason, isolation with rubber dam is essential. A wooden wedge should be placed interdentally to retract the rubber gingivally, preventing it from being cut with the bur. The wedge will move the teeth apart slightly, which helps to establish a tight contact point when the restoration is placed. This technique is called *pre-wedging*.

Aspects of cavity preparation

The cavity preparation is identical with that described previously (Fig. 7.11(a)). Access is gained to carious dentine by removing sufficient enamel over it to allow access to the enamel–dentine junction. All caries is removed from the enamel–dentine junction and soft caries excavated over the pulp.

It is principally in the management of the cavity margin that the preparation for receiving a composite may differ from that for filling with amalgam. Two aspects merit discussion:

- What should be done with undermined enamel? Can it be left and supported by composite or must it be removed?

- How should the enamel margins be finished? Should they be bevelled to increase the area available for retention and improve marginal seal, or should they be finished to a butt joint as in the amalgam restoration (Fig. 7.11(a))?

There are currently no hard and fast rules as to how to answer either question because insufficient clinical research has been carried out. However, it is probably better to err on the side of a conservative approach and leave, rather than remove, unsupported enamel.

The question of bevelling provokes particular controversy. Some prepare the cavity exactly as if it were to receive an amalgam restoration. Others place a small bevel occlusally and gingivally and long bevels on the axial enamel walls. This cavity design has been called the *adhesive cavity preparation*.

Lining and etching the cavity

Before the enamel cavity walls are etched with phosphoric acid, all exposed dentine should be protected. A proprietary cement containing calcium hydroxide is suitable (Fig. 7.11(b)), but zinc oxide and eugenol materials must not be used because they inhibit the polymerization of the composite resin. Calcium hydroxide should always be used in a deep cavity, as discussed on p. 65, together with a further thick lining of glass ionomer cement.

Fig. 7.11 (*right*) (a) Cavity prepared in a lower premolar for a posterior composite restoration. Approximal caries and occlusal caries were removed. The occlusal caries was found to be minimal and the cavity was not extended into dentine. Note the wedge separating the teeth to facilitate the establishment of a contact point.
(b) A proprietary cement containing calcium hydroxide is used to line the exposed dentine.
(c) The enamel walls are etched with phosphoric acid gel.
(d) The acid gel is washed away and the enamel dried. A strip or mylar matrix is wedged in position with a light-reflecting wedge.
(e) The bonding resin is applied and light cured.
(f) The first portion of composite is placed cervically and polymerized with light directed from the buccal side along the wedge.
(g) The final increment of composite is contoured as much as possible before it is polymerized.
(h) A multibladed tungsten carbide finishing bur is used to contour the marginal ridge. The mylar matrix has been removed but a metal matrix could be left in place while this is done to protect the adjacent tooth.
(i) An abrasive disc is used to smooth the marginal ridge.
(j) Occlusally, alumina-impregnated rubber points can be used to smooth the restoration.
(k) The completed restoration before removing the rubber dam and checking the occlusion.

(a)

(b)

(c)

(d)

(e)

(f)

(g)

(h)

(i)

(j)

(k)

The advantages of extending a layer of the glass ionomer lining material over the cervical floor are as follows:

- The material adheres to enamel and dentine, and composite adheres to it, to some extent.

- It is a permanent restorative material and is produced in radiopaque and light-curing forms which are visible on radiographs. This is essential if any subsequent secondary caries is to be diagnosed radiographically (see p. 184).

- It contains fluoride and is thus cariostatic and may protect the vulnerable cervical floor of the restoration from secondary caries.

- Although glass ionomer cement is currently not strong enough to resist occlusal stress, it will be covered by a posterior composite resin which is considerably stronger in this respect.

- The layered restoration may in some ways be regarded as replacement of dentine by glass ionomer cement and replacement of enamel by composite resin, with the bond between the two being analogous to the enamel–dentine junction.

Once the lining material has been placed, the enamel walls are etched with phosphoric acid (Fig. 7.11(c)). It is not advisable to etch the glass ionomer current to improve its bond with the composite. Autocuring materials will be damaged by the etchant. However, the newer light-curing resin-modified glass ionomer materials will form a chemical bond with the composite resin. Thus the enamel walls of the cavity should be etched and the area thoroughly washed and dried (Fig. 7.11(d)).

Placing the matrix and restoration

Although the composite resins made for use in posterior teeth are viscous, they are still not viscous enough to be positively condensed into the cavity in the same way as amalgam. For this reason, the approximal contour of the final restoration will be dictated by the shape of the matrix. Forming a tight contact area is difficult with these materials.

Pre-wedging, as described on p. 126, is helpful. A thin matrix should be chosen which may be metal or clear mylar strip or pre-contoured plastic. Metal has the advantage that it can be firmly burnished against the adjacent tooth. Mylar strip has the advantage that the curing light can shine through it. When the cavity is small a retainer is not essential, and in a tooth where only one approximal surface is involved in the cavity it is sensible not to pass a band around the tooth. The thickness of the band in the uncut contact area will move the tooth slightly, thus partly negating the pre-wedging effect.

Once the band is in position, it must be firmly wedged cervically. Light-reflecting wedges are now available for use with light-cured materials (Fig. 7.11(d)). These wedges are designed to reflect the light at right angles to the wedge to polymerize the critical cervical margin of the restoration. The cavity is now ready for the application of the bonding agent and the composite material. The bonding agent is mixed and applied to the dried surface with a disposable brush (Fig. 7.11(e)) and air blown gently to ensure a thin film. It is particularly important to avoid gingival pooling of the bonding resin. The bonding resin is light cured.

The composite is now placed, in increments if necessary, starting at the deepest portion of the cavity (Fig. 7.11(f)). Where a light-reflecting wedge is used the first increment is polymerized with light directed from the buccal or lingual side. This will ensure the proper polymerization of the resin in a very confined area as well as minimizing the polymerization contraction of the resin. A Teflon-coated instrument with smooth rounded ends, is a useful packing instrument. If packed incrementally, each increment is light cured before the next is added. No increment should exceed 2.0–2.5 mm in depth.

As the composite approaches the cavo-surface margin it should be contoured to a reasonable anatomical form, thus minimizing the need for removal of gross excess during finishing (Fig. 7.11(g)).

Finishing the restoration

While the matrix band is still in place, excess material is removed from the occlusal embrasure area with a multibladed tungsten carbide bur or coarse composite finishing diamond bur at high speed (Fig. 7.11(h)). At the same time the shape of the marginal ridge area is established using the band as a guard for the approximal surface of the adjacent tooth.

The matrix band and wedge are then removed and excess is removed from the approximal and occlusal surfaces using the same bur. A tapered white stone or finer composite finishing diamond bur can be used to accentuate the occlusal anatomy. Where possible, a series of abrasive discs are used to smooth the restoration (Fig. 7.11(i)), but occlusally, where these discs will not fit the contours of the tooth, alumina-impregnated rubber points can be used (Figs. 7.11 (j) and 7.11(k)). Finally, the wedge is removed and the contact point checked with floss.

Once the rubber dam is removed, the occlusion should be checked with articulating paper and adjusted as necessary.

APPROXIMAL 'ADHESIVE' RESTORATIONS: MARGINAL RIDGE PRESERVED

Up to now consideration has been given to cavity preparation where the marginal ridge has been removed to gain access to the carious dentine cervical to it. Since caries has undermined the marginal ridge, this is an obvious approach. However, this access is unnecessarily destructive in small cavities and an approach may be made occlusally or buccally, preserving the marginal ridge (Fig. 7.12(a)). This approach has been made possible by the adhesive materials (glass ionomer cement and composite resin). Nevertheless, caries should not be treated operatively at any earlier stage to facilitate this approach because an arrested enamel lesion is still preferable to a restoration, however small.

Occlusal approach

Having applied rubber dam, a small round bur in the airotor handpiece is used to enter the occlusal side of the marginal ridge, directing the bur diagonally towards the caries (Figs. 7.12(b) and 3.3). The orifice of the cavity should be wide enough bucco-lingually to obtain adequate visibility and access to the carious dentine beneath. Caries is removed from the enamel–dentine junction with a round bur. The resulting cavity will present two holes in the enamel, one occlusally cut by the dentist and one approximally resulting from caries. It is therefore sometimes called a 'tunnel' cavity or an 'internal' cavity preparation.

A thin soft metal matrix is contoured and wedged firmly in position. If the cavity is deep, the dentine nearest the pulp is covered with a thin layer of a proprietary cement containing calcium hydroxide. The polyacrylic acid conditioning agent supplied with the glass ionomer cement should now be applied to the cavity with a brush or small pledget of cotton-wool. After 10 seconds the cavity is throughly washed and dried.

A strongly radiopaque glass ionomer material containing silver particles (cermet), produced in capsule form, is mixed, the capsule is inserted into the applicator, and the material is syringed into the cavity (Fig. 7.12(c)). Excess material is left on the surface and this can be removed, after it has set, with a multibladed tungsten carbide bur in the airotor. Alternatively a radio-opaque resin-modified glass ionomer cement

Fig. 7.12 (a) Clinical examination shows obvious occlusal caries in this lower first molar. A bite-wing radiograph (Fig. 7.1) shows approximal lesions, involving dentine.
(b) Occlusal caries has been removed and the cavity extended distally and bucco-lingually to allow a round bur access to the approximal caries. A proprietary cement containing calcium hydroxide has been used to line the deep portion of the cavity, and a thin soft metal matrix has been wedged firmly into position. A similar cavity has been prepared on the mesial aspect of the tooth.
(c) A radiopaque glass ionomer material, containing silver particles, (cermet) is syringed into the cavity, having used the polyacrylic acid conditioning agent supplied with the material.
(d) The occlusal portion of the glass ionomer cement is removed with an airotor and the enamel walls are acid etched, washed, and dried.
(e) The occlusal cavities are filled with a light-cured posterior composite resin.

(a)

(b)

(c)

(d)

(e)

can be chosen, encapsulated, and syringed in the same manner. The material should be firmly tamped into position to ensure good adaptation within the cavity. The set of this material is initiated by light curing.

Once the glass ionomer has set, the occlusal portion is removed with the airotor (Fig. 7.12(d)). The enamel walls can now be etched and a posterior composite placed in the occlusal surface (Fig. 7.12(e)).

Buccal approach

This approach is particularly well suited to teeth which are tilted lingually, where an occlusal approach to caries would result in the removal of considerable sound tooth substance, or where mesial or distal tilting has produced an unusual contact area down towards the cement–enamel junction. However, a buccal approach to caries destroys the buccal wall of the cavity, and if the marginal ridge collapses during cavity preparation, retention will be lost. Therefore careful judgement of the strength of the marginal ridge is important before choosing this design. Access to caries is gained with a small round bur in the airotor and caries is removed from the enamel–dentine junction with a small round bur at slow speed. Since the cavity is not subject to occlusal stress, undermined enamel may be left provided that the dentist can see or feel the enamel–dentine junction with a probe to check that it is caries-free (Figs. 7.13 and 3.3).

Fig. 7.13 A buccal approach to approximal caries in a lingually tilted lower premolar. Any occlusal approach would be unnecessarily difficult and destructive of sound tooth tissue in this situation.

The cavity is lined and filled as described in the previous section, except that after insertion of the filling material, the matrix is pulled firmly around the tooth to assist the contouring of the restoration. Where a light cured material is used, the matrix strip should be made of mylar or polyester so that the light can shine through it to polymerize the filling material. Since this restoration takes no occlusal load, replacement of part of the glass ionomer material by the composite resin is not usually necessary.

Approximal root caries

Root caries presents some specific operative difficulties relating to access and retention of the restoration. When the lesion is very superficial, it may be possible to smooth and polish the carious area without needing to place a restoration. If the lesion has penetrated more deeply, a restoration will usually be required to aid plaque control and protect the pulp.

Since the caries is on the approximal surface of the root, it would be very destructive to approach it through the marginal ridge. Buccal access is often the most convenient approach although if the lesion were sited more to the lingual side, access from this direction could be preferable. Caries is removed with round burs in the low-speed handpiece until the periphery of the cavity is caries-free. Where the handpiece head obstructs vision an excavator with a long shank can be useful, because it may be easier to see the caries as it is being removed.

Once the periphery of the cavity is judged to be hard, soft dentine caries over the pulpal surface should be removed. Particular care must be taken not to expose the pulp traumatically, since the pulp chamber or root canal are soon reached.

The cavity is lined with a proprietary cement containing calcium hydroxide and filled with a radiopaque glass ionomer cement or cermet. Since this is adhesive to dentine, mechanical retention in the form of an undercut cavity is not required, but the polyacrylic acid conditioning agent supplied with the material should always be used to ensure an optimum bond.

THE MESIAL–OCCLUSAL–DISTAL [MOD] CAVITY

So far the cavities described have been on one *or* other approximal surface, with or without the inclusion of the occlusal surface. Therefore the restorations are described as follows:

- mesial
- distal
- mesial–occlusal (MO)
- distal–occlusal (DO).

Commonly, when circumstances favour the initiation of caries, lesions occur on both the mesial and distal surfaces of the same tooth. They can be restored separately by mesial and distal fillings or in some cases by separate MO and DO fillings. This is often done in upper molar teeth, preserving the oblique ridge and thereby more of the strength of the tooth (Fig. 4.18).

However, it is often necessary to join the cavities producing a mesial–occlusal–distal (MOD) cavity. The preparation does not differ much from the MO or DO cavity except that the natural shape of the cavity makes it easy to produce a retentive design. There is more difficulty in ensuring that the other aspects of the design are right. The approximal boxes should be retentive in their own right so that the occlusal part of the cavity can be kept as narrow as possible commensurate with removing the caries; overcutting the occlusal part of the cavity is likely to result in cusp fracture at a later date. It may be that, with further development, the layered restoration, with a glass ionomer base and an occlusal surface in composite which bonds to enamel thus splinting the cusps together, is a solution to this problem.

The matrix for an MOD amalgam restoration is similar to an MO or DO except that even more care is needed, since the effect of burnishing the band against one contact point may be to pull it away from the other. The answer is to rely on the wedges to achieve cervical adaptation and slacken the band a little.

Removing the band is also more difficult, but the other stages are similar to the MO or DO restoration.

PROBLEMS OF THE LARGER CAVITY

Large restorations may be required either as a result of untreated or recurrent caries or because repeated replacement of restorations has, over a period of years, undermined the strength of the occlusal surface. The principles underlying the restoration of the badly broken-down tooth are the same as those already discussed for smaller restorations. However, these teeth present certain specific difficulties which will now be discussed.

Pre-operative assessment

Changes in the pulp are more likely with large lesions, and a full assessment of the condition of the pulp should be made, including vitality tests, and any necessary root treatment provided before the definitive restoration of the tooth is placed.

Clinical examination will give an idea of the extent of the caries and/or existing restorations and their relationship to the gingival margin. Where caries is well subgingival, periodontal surgery may be required before the tooth is finally restored. This involves reflecting buccal and lingual flaps. The relation of the base of the cavity to the height of the alveolar bone will then be obvious. It may be necessary to remove alveolar bone so that some sound root remains apical to the cavity. The flaps are then sutured so that the base of the cavity will be just supragingival.

The occlusion should be examined in the intercuspal position and in lateral excursions. Problems such as over-eruption of an opposing tooth may then be anticipated. The dentist may elect to re-contour the opposing tooth before restoring the broken-down tooth.

Both bite-wing and periapical radiographs should be examined. The bite-wing radiograph can be used to assess the size of the carious lesion and/or an existing restoration, its proximity to the pulp, and its relationship to the alveolar bone (Fig. 7.14(a)). The periapical radiograph may reveal a periapical radiolucency (Fig. 7.14(b)), showing that root canal treatment is required if the tooth is to be saved. The periapical radiograph will also show the number and curvature of roots and root canals and their patency, all of which will be important if root canal treatment is required.

With a vital pulp, bacterial contamination from saliva should be avoided. Rubber dam should be used and wedges should be placed to retract the rubber and prevent it from being snagged by a bur (Fig. 7.15(a)).

Caries removal

Access to carious dentine is gained by removing any remaining enamel over it with the airotor. Old restorations are removed (see p. 186), taking care not to cut away sound tooth substance (Fig. 7.15(b)). The enamel–dentine junction is made caries-free with a round bur at low speed. Where enamel undermined by caries prevents access to the enamel–dentine junction, some of the undermined enamel should be removed (Fig. 7.15(c)).

(a)

(b)

Fig. 7.14 (a) A bite-wing radiograph showing a large distal cavity in the upper first premolar. There is also occlusal caries in the lower molar. (b) A periapical radiograph of the same tooth showing a periapical area.

Finally, caries over the pulp is removed. Since demineralization of dentine precedes bacterial penetration, stained but firm dentine may be left over the pulp where it is thought that its removal might result in pulp exposure. Exposures that are too small to be seen (micro-exposures) may be present in the depth of the cavity and so deep parts of the cavity should always be covered with a proprietary lining containing calcium hydroxide (indirect pulp cap). Where a frank carious exposure is found immediately beneath soft caries, root canal treatment or possibly extraction is

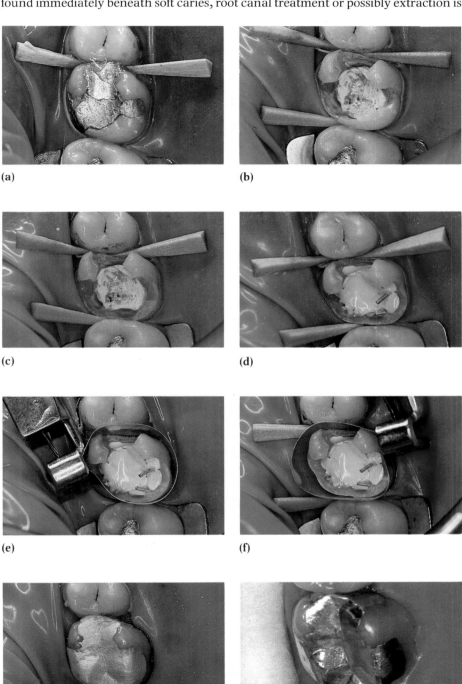

(a)

(b)

(c)

(d)

(e)

(f)

(g)

(h)

Fig. 7.15   (a) The amalgam in this heavily restored upper first molar is to be replaced. The patient has noticed some discomfort with hot and cold. The tooth is vital and there is no periapical area. A local anaesthetic has been given and a rubber dam placed.
(b) The old restoration is removed. There is caries beneath the enamel–dentine junction distally, but the old lining is left in place because this is a deep cavity and there is no evidence of active caries beneath the lining.
(c) Removal of caries at the enamel–dentine junction distally necessitates removal of overhanging enamel in this area. Loss of this tissue leaves few retentive features in this cavity preparation. For this reason, pins are required.
(d) Three pins are placed to aid retention of the amalgam. They are positioned distobuccally, distopalatally, and palatally. A proprietary lining containing calcium hydroxide is placed.
(e) A badly placed matrix. There is no room for amalgam between the distobuccal pin and the matrix band.
(f) The matrix band is reapplied with the retainer lingually. There is now room for amalgam around all the pins and the contact points are burnished. Wedges are in place to prevent an excess of amalgam cervically.
(g) The band is removed and the amalgam carved. The rubber dam must now be removed and the occlusion checked.
(h) At a subsequent visit the amalgam is polished. Note that blue articulating paper has been used to show that this restoration is in occlusion!

indicated becáuse the prognosis for the pulp is poor even if there have been no symptoms. Occasionally, calcium hydroxide is used as a direct pulp cap over a small pulp exposure in a symptomless vital tooth when the exposure results from removing the last bit of firm caries. Exclusion of saliva from the cavity may be important to preserving a healthy vital pulp in these cases. However, root canal treatment is usually required because pulp capping may be followed by chronic pulpitis.

Designing the restoration

Thus far the design of the cavity has been dictated entirely by the extent of the caries and any previous restorations. It is now time to put down the handpiece and think about the eventual restoration.

If root canal treatment is required, this is best carried out through some form of temporary restoration, usually glass ionomer cement. Once root canal treatment is complete, restoration of the crown can be undertaken.

The relationship of the gingival floor of the cavity to the gingival margin must be assessed. Occasionally, caries results in the margin of the restoration being apical to the crest of the alveolar bone. In these cases, periodontal surgery and removal of some alveolar bone is essential before the tooth can be restored permanently. However, if the margin is just within the gingival crevice, a permanent restoration can be inserted provided that rubber dam is used to prevent contamination of the filling material with blood, saliva, or crevicular fluid.

Choice of restorative material

The strength of the remaining tooth tissue must be assessed. Undermined enamel in areas of occlusal stress will eventually have to be removed. A decision must be taken as to whether the remaining tooth structure is strong enough to support a restoration, or whether it is weak and must be supported *by* the restoration. Figure 7.16 shows a first premolar and a molar where the enamel and dentine are strong enough to support amalgam restorations.

However, the cusps of the second premolar have been weakened and, although they are still supported by dentine, they are liable to fracture under occlusal stress. In this tooth, a cast metal restoration should be considered to protect the remaining tooth tissue (see Chapter 10).

It is possible to replace or cover weak cusps with amalgam, but an adequate bulk of amalgam (a minimum of 3 mm in height) must be used and this reduction of cusp height produces retention problems.

Figures 6.4(a)–6.4(i) show an occlusal cavity where the remaining tooth tissue is weak. This cavity, which is completely enclosed in enamel, may best be restored by using adhesive restorative materials which bond to and support the dental tissues. In this case, after placing a layer of a proprietary cement containing calcium hydroxide, the missing dentine was replaced with glass ionomer cement. Then a posterior composite was placed after the enamel walls had been acid etched (see Chapter 6). The main disadvantage of this approach is the relatively large area of occlusal composite, which is likely to wear away. There is also the danger that the composite may cause wear of the opposing tooth. Further possible approaches being evaluated clinically are to use composite resin inlays, cured outside the mouth and then cemented, or, alternatively, porcelain inlays (see p. 173).

The following list summarizes the current choice of restorative material and the type of preparation for a badly broken-down posterior tooth:

- amalgam retained by undercuts and other intracoronal retentive features
- amalgam retained by pins
- posterior composite

Fig. 7.16 Old amalgam restorations and caries have been removed from three teeth. The first premolar and first molar have cusps judged to be strong enough to support amalgam restorations. However, the cusps of the second premolar are weaker and consideration is given to using cast metal to protect the remaining tooth tissue.

- a glass ionomer and posterior composite layered restoration
- a cast metal inlay with cusp protection
- a glass ionomer or composite restoration with a laboratory processed porcelain or composite resin occlusal surface
- a core of pin-retained amalgam, pin- or acid-etch-retained composite, or glass ionomer, supporting a crown.

The first five options are considered here; the sixth is a possible option which is still in the developmental stage and the final option, the provision of crowns, is beyond the scope of this book.

Pin retention for large restorations and cores

Badly broken-down teeth frequently present problems of retention which are solved by the use of corrosion-resistant pins. Part of the pin is inserted into the dentine while the remainder protrudes into the cavity to be surrounded by the restorative material—often amalgam. Where a large amount of tooth is missing, the number, position, and angle of the pins must be carefully planned. The principle is that it should not be possible to dislodge the restoration in any of the five directions (buccally, lingually, mesially, distally, or occlusally) or at any angle between them. For example, one pin, if it is at an angle to one of the cavity walls, will prevent both occlusal and lateral displacement, but if it cannot be inserted at an angle to a cavity wall, thus creating an undercut, then two pins at an angle to each other will be needed. Often the application of these principles results in one pin being placed for each missing cusp. Thus, where a lingual or buccal wall is missing, two pins might be used. However, one pin per cusp is *not* a firm rule (Fig. 7.15(d)). It is a mistake to use more pins than absolutely necessary because they weaken both the tooth and the restoration. However, where a core is being made to support a crown, additional pins may be required to take account of the loss of retention which sometimes results when more tooth tissue is removed in the crown preparation. The operator should mentally superimpose the crown preparation before deciding how many pins are required.

The pin-hole should be placed in the greatest bulk of dentine available, but never in the enamel and never at the enamel–dentine junction, as the undermined enamel would break away. Pin-holes should be 2–2.5 mm deep, with the diameter ranging from 0.5 to 0.7 mm according to the make of pin.

Three types of pin are used: cemented pins slightly smaller then the hole prepared for them, smooth friction-retained pins pressed into holes slightly smaller than the pin, and self-tapping threaded pins. The last of those is the most convenient and retentive, and so only this type will be described.

Pin kits are available consisting of a twist drill with a shoulder to control the depth of penetration and a matched self-tapping threaded pin (Fig. 7.17). When preparing the pin-hole the twist drill must be rotating clockwise, otherwise it will not cut. A low-speed handpiece is used, and it should have good bearings so that the drill does not waver in the head of the handpiece and produce an oversized hole.

The pin must be placed in the dentine and should not perforate either the pulp or the periodontal membrane. When in doubt about the angulation of the pin it is helpful to place a flat plastic instrument gently down the outside of the root. A pin-hole prepared parallel to this should not perforate either the pulp or the periodontal membrane.

The twist drill is inserted to the shoulder and then removed. The dental nurse should blow away the dentine dust so that the operator can see. The twist drill should never be stalled while cutting the hole because this usually results in breaking the drill. The pin is supplied attached to a disposable latch bur shank, and

Fig. 7.17 A twist drill with a matched, self-tapping, threaded pin.

the low-speed handpiece is used to thread the pin into the hole. It shears at a notch 2–3 mm above the dentine surface.

It is sometimes necessary to shorten the pin with a diamond bur in the airotor because amalgam 1 mm thick should cover the pin in the finished restoration. Where a crown is to be prepared, the operator should once again mentally superimpose the preparation to ensure that amalgam will remain around the pin after the crown has been prepared. It is sometimes necessary to bend the pin inwards to ensure that it will be surrounded by amalgam after crown preparation.

Occasionally, the pulp may be perforated when a pin-hole is being prepared. If this happens, a proprietary cement containing calcium hydroxide should be placed gently down the pin-hole with a probe. If symptoms of pulpitis develop or if the pulp becomes necrotic, root canal therapy will be required. If the periodontal membrane is perforated by a pin, it is usually necessary to extend the cavity margin to include the defect. Alternatively, a radiopaque glass ionomer cement can be used to fill the defect.

Placing the matrix, packing, carving, and finishing

Placing a matrix can be one of the most difficult parts of restoring a badly broken-down tooth. The time taken to achieve a good matrix is well spent, however, because this is critical to the success of the operation.

When placing the matrix it is easy to trap the rubber dam between the matrix band and the tooth. The rubber should be pulled firmly out of the way when placing the band to avoid this.

In an attempt to achieve a stable matrix system it is tempting to overtighten the band around the tooth. This may result in a defective contact point or insufficient room for amalgam between the pins and the band (Fig. 7.15(e)). One way round this problem is to use a matrix system in the form of a band with a tightening screw, but no retainer. The band is sufficiently curved to grip the tooth cervically while flaring out occlusally (Fig. 7.9). An alternative solution to the problem is to use a carefully wedged conventional matrix retainer and band (Fig. 7.15(f)), possibly stabilizing it in position with composition.

The matrix band must be slightly higher than the highest cusp to be replaced. It is particularly easy to misjudge this with upper premolar teeth where the cusp tip is well coronal to the marginal ridge.

The help of a dental nurse when placing the amalgam is invaluable. More than one mix of amalgam will be required and a new mix should not be prepared until the operator is ready for it. If this procedure is not observed, the operator will be handling the alloy when it is past its working time. In many dental schools it is currently considered economically unrealistic for dental students to work with a dental nurse at all times. However, when placing a large restoration such assistance is almost mandatory.

Initially, amalgam should be firmly condensed around the pins, taking care to pack amalgam between the pins and the matrix band. The amalgam should cover the pins and finally be overpacked.

Carving is carried out as described previously, with as much as possible being carried out before the matrix band is removed. Once the band is removed, particular care should be taken to ensure that there is no ledge of amalgam cervically (Fig. 7.15(g)). When the rubber dam has been removed, the occlusion is checked with articulating paper and shimstock, and the patient is warned to bite very gently initially. The restoration is finally smoothed with cotton-wool and the patient is asked to avoid chewing hard on that side for a few hours.

The amalgam can be polished at a subsequent appointment (Fig. 7.15(h)). A carefully executed pinned amalgam restoration can serve for many years provided that further caries is prevented.

FURTHER READING

Mount, G. J. (1994). *An atlas of glass-ionomer cements. A clinician's guide* (2nd edn). Martin Dunitz, London.

Wilson, A. D. and McLean, J. W. (1988). *Glass ionomer cements.* Quintessence, Chicago, IL.

Winstanley, R. B. (1983). Pinned retention—10 years on. *Dent. Update* 10, 246–52.

8 Treatment of smooth surface caries, erosion—abrasion lesions, and enamel hypoplasia

SMOOTH SURFACE ENAMEL CARIES

The buccal pit of lower molar teeth, the palatal groove of upper molars, and the cingulum pits of upper incisor teeth are plaque stagnation areas and are susceptible to caries in the same way as the occlusal fissures. However, enamel caries occurring elsewhere on the buccal or lingual surfaces is usually a sign of a high caries rate and poor oral hygiene. These areas are the easiest to keep clean, and caries can be prevented here by good oral hygiene, even in the absence of other preventive measures. This means that when initial enamel lesions occur on the buccal or lingual surfaces the chances are that there will be extensive caries elsewhere in the mouth and the major emphasis must be on prevention.

With poor oral hygiene, plaque accumulates beneath the maximum bulbosity of the teeth where it is protected from abrasion by cheeks and tongue. This may occur in both arches. Therefore smooth surface enamel caries is most common around the necks of the molar and premolar teeth and on the labio-cervical surfaces of the incisors (Fig. 8.1). Caries is rare on the palatal surface of the upper incisor teeth, other than in cingulum pits, and enamel caries is extremely rare on the lingual surface of the lower incisors. It is less common on the labial surface of lower incisors than upper incisors. When there has been a degree of gingival recession, caries often starts at the cement-enamel junction, undermining the enamel.

Where enamel caries is diagnosed at the stage of the white spot lesion, i.e. before cavitation occurs, preventive measures should be used to arrest the lesion. Restoration is indicated only where there is a cavity that hinders plaque control or the pulp is endangered.

ROOT CARIES

Dentine caries on the root of a tooth following gingival recession has a number of characteristics which distinguish it from other types of caries (see Chapter 1, p. 8). It does not need to penetrate enamel and often starts over a large area of the root. It is often circumferential and there may be no distinction between approximal, buccal, and lingual lesions. It is predominantly a disease of older people, because gingival recession is more common in this group, but it may occur in younger age groups if roots are exposed. It is sometimes continuous, with caries at the cement-enamel junction undermining the enamel, but does not always spread apically as the gingival margin recedes. New lesions may develop later at the level of the new gingival margin.

(a)

(b)

(c)

(d)

(e)

(f)

Fig. 8.1 (a) Caries at the gingival margin of the lower canine tooth.
(b) A lesion isolated with a rubber dam using a clamp to retract the gingival margin sufficiently to expose the entire lesion.
(c) Caries has been removed with a steel bur at low speed. There are no natural undercuts but enamel is still present gingivally.
(d) Cavity lined with calcium hydroxide lining material.
(e) Acid-etching gel placed.
(f) The restored tooth immediately after the removal of the rubber dam.

Clinically, both active and slowly progressing or arrested lesions can be seen. Active lesions are soft, close to the gingival margin, whereas arrested or slowly progressing lesions are harder and are apparently left abandoned by receding gingival margins in patients with progressive periodontal disease.

Prevention is very important in the management of root caries but may be difficult because it often arises in older people who are having problems in maintaining previously good levels of oral hygiene. In addition, older people are frequently taking medicines which depress salivary flow and this xerostomia makes dental caries more likely. Tranquillizers, antidepressants, antihypertensives, and diuretics all have a xerostomic effect. The feeling of a dry mouth may be alleviated by sucking sweets or taking frequent drinks, many of which are cariogenic. Finally, retirement, bereavement, or illness may result in dietary changes which favour caries.

Early diagnosis is very important so that the dentist can help the patient to find the cause of the root caries and prevent its progression. Plaque control, dietary advice, and topical fluorides are all important in the management of the disease. The aim should be to *arrest* the early lesion so that, over time, a soft area of active root caries becomes hard.

Smoothing and polishing the softened root surface may sometimes assist plaque control and favour lesion arrest. Such areas do not require restorations unless there is an aesthetic problem.

However, a cavitated lesion may endanger the pulp, may be sensitive, and hinders plaque control. In these cases a restoration is indicated.

RESTORATION OF FREE SMOOTH SURFACE CARIOUS LESIONS [BOTH ENAMEL AND ROOT CARIES]

Access to caries

Compared with the lesions described in Chapters 6 and 7, access is much easier. Some lesions affect a wide surface area and problems of access are associated with the surrounding structures rather than the lesions themselves. Access to cervical caries on the buccal surface of upper second and third molars is hindered by the coronoid process of the mandible when the mouth is opened widely. This is a common site for caries because access for the toothbrush is also restricted. A miniature handpiece head and miniature burs may be used, and it is easier to position the head of the handpiece if these lesions are treated with the mouth partly closed.

There is a similar problem with access to the lingual surface of the lower molar teeth when the tongue is large and active. The problem here is mainly to keep a dry field. Rubber dam can be difficult to place. If it is possible to get the rubber dam down below the lesion, it should be placed over teeth right around to the other side of the arch so that the rubber is stretched away from the lingual surface of the tooth to be treated. If it comes straight up from the lingual side of the clamp, it obstructs the handpiece head. If a rubber dam cannot be placed, a large flanged saliva ejector can be used to aspirate saliva, retract the tongue, and retract and protect the floor of the mouth (see Figs. 4.8 and 8.2).

Fig. 8.2 A flanged saliva injector in place. This retracts and protects the tongue and floor of the mouth. Its polished surface also acts as a mirror and can help the dentist to see.

Removal of caries

In removing enamel caries on smooth surfaces it is often difficult to know where to start and where to stop. The following will help the decision.

• The white or brown spot lesion can be arrested by preventive means (plaque control; fluoride application in the form of toothpaste, mouthrinse, or varnish; dietary analysis and advice) and a restoration is not required.

• The rationale for restorative management, in addition to prevention, is to restore the integrity of the tooth surface to aid plaque control and protect the pulp.

Thus, caries removal should start in the area of cavitation and the preparation can often be done with round steel burs in the low-speed handpiece (Figs. 8.1(b) and 8.1(c)). The white spot lesion will often extend widely around the tooth, sometimes including the approximal surface, but if the area has not cavitated it should not normally be removed.

Similarly, in removing root caries it is often difficult to know where to stop. Often large areas of the root surface are discoloured or softened. Soft dentine should be removed, but hard stained dentine can be left even when it is adjacent to an area which is to be restored. There is a temptation to feel that while one is restoring the tooth it might be as well to tidy up the whole of the affected area, but this can lead to very large cavities which are difficult, if not impossible, to restore.

When using a round bur to remove carious dentine on the root surface the bur should be kept at about 45° to the tooth surface, because the side of the bur cuts more efficiently than the end. Since these lesions are often circumferential this will mean continually reorientating the head of the handpiece. It is possible to improve control of the handpiece by guiding the head of the handpiece with the left hand (right hand for left-handed operators). It is important to remember not to cut too deeply because the root canal is easily exposed. This is particularly likely in root caries because reparative dentine forms at the pulpal ends of the affected tubules. Since the tubules run cervically in this area, reparative dentine is more apically placed than might be expected.

Choice of restorative material

Once the caries has been removed there is often a wide shallow cavity with no natural undercuts (Fig. 8.1(c)). The following restorative materials can be used:

- composite resin

- glass ionomer cement or cermet.

When all the walls of the cavity are in enamel an acid-etch-retained composite is a logical choice. Further cavity preparation is not needed unless an additional area is thought necessary for acid-etch retention. In this case, the enamel margins can be bevelled, and this bevelling also has the effect of blending the appearance of the composite restoration into the remainder of the enamel. A composite resin is a particularly good choice where appearance is important, and in this case a microfine filled material would be chosen because the smaller filler particles (0.4 μm silica particles) allow the material to be polished.

In root caries the material of choice will usually be a glass ionomer cement or cermet because it is adhesive to dentine and releases fluoride which has a cariostatic effect. Composite is not ideal because there is no enamel available for acid-etched retention. Amalgam should not be used because it is difficult to cut retentive cavities where there are large circumferential lesions, without seriously weakening the tooth and it has no cariostatic properties which are particularly important with root caries.

Where the cavity has a cervical margin on dentine and an occlusal margin on enamel, glass ionomer and composite can be combined in a layered technique (Fig. 8.3). Glass ionomer cement replaces the dentine, and subsequently a composite resin replaces the enamel. This layered restoration combines the adhesive and cariostatic properties of glass ionomer cement with the good appearance and wear characteristics of composite resin. When using auto-cure glass ionomer cements the cavity should initially be completely restored with glass ionomer material. At a subsequent visit a layer of glass ionomer cement is removed and the enamel exposed. This enamel and the surface of the glass ionomer is now etched for 15 seconds before placing the bonding resin and finally the composite material.

If a resin-modified glass ionomer cement is used for this layered technique, it is possible to place both the glass ionomer and the composite materials at the same visit. Initially the glass ionomer is placed and light cured. The cavity is now redeveloped in the cement to allow sufficient room for a laminate of composite resin. Sound enamel walls are exposed to allow use of the acid-etch technique. With a resin-modified glass ionomer cement it is only necessary to etch the enamel wall since these cements contain sufficient free radicals in the resin component to obtain a chemical union.

Lining

Deep carious cavities, particularly in young patients, should be lined with a calcium hydroxide lining material (Fig. 8.1 (d)). In cavities to be filled with composite resin, the dentine should be protected before the enamel is acid etched.

(a)

(b)

(c)

(e)

Fig. 8.3 (a) Secondary caries at the cervical margin of the restoration in the upper lateral incisor.
(b) After removing the old restoration and caries the exposed dentine has been lined with glass ionomer cement and the incisal enamel cavity margin bevelled. Excess cement cervically has been removed with a bur.
(c) Acid-etching gel being applied with a brush. The gel is left for only 15 seconds to avoid damaging the structure of the glass ionomer cement.
(d) The etched enamel.
(e) The restoration is completed by adding a layer of composite. (By courtesy of Messrs A. C. Shortall, R. L. Baylor, and J. R. Grundy. Reproduced from *Restorative Dentistry* by permission of A. E. Morgan Publications Ltd.)

Applying the matrix and placing the restoration

Composite resin

Initially, the operator must decide which composite is to be used. The selection will involve the following:

- Deciding whether a microfine, conventional, or hybrid material is to be used. Microfine materials have the best appearance but conventional or hybrid materials have better wear characteristics.

- Deciding whether the material will be chemically cured or light cured. The latter group have the advantage of a longer working time and are thus favoured in more complex cavities and indeed have now virtually replaced chemically cured composites for the majority of restorations. They should be cured in increments no thicker than 2 mm, and so larger restorations should be built up in layers with a thick glass ionomer base leaving less than 2 mm thickness to be filled by the composite.

- Deciding the shade using the shade guide supplied by the manufacturer.

When using a light-cured material the layer of bonding resin is light cured before applying the composite. If the cavity is no deeper than 2 mm, the entire restoration can be placed and contoured before curing. The working time is not unlimited because the material begins to set under the operating light. To prevent this, either the operating light should be switched off or a protective filter should be inserted between the light and the tooth.

Most dentists insert these restorations free-hand, but if a matrix is required a cellulose acetate type, which will allow the light to pass through it, should be chosen. These matrices have small handles which allow them to be placed with tweezers.

An alternative matrix is a contoured mylar strip which is wrapped around the tooth, passing through both contact points. It is then pulled up against the gingival margin of the preparation contouring the restorative material cervically. Any excess is left on the occlusal side of the cavity, and this can be removed once the material has set.

Glass ionomer cement

The dentine conditioning agent supplied with the material (10 per cent polyacrylic acid) should be applied to the cavity for 10 seconds and then the cavity should be thoroughly washed and dried. Auto-cure (chemically set) glass ionomer cement restorations are usually placed with a matrix. The matrix protects the material while it is setting and should contour it so that minimal finishing is required.

Before placing the filling, the appropriate size of metal matrix should be burnished with a metal flat plastic to fit the tooth. The flat plastic can then be warmed in a flame, dipped into sticky wax, and then replaced on the matrix. This attaches the matrix to the flat plastic and makes it easier to re-position it accurately onto the tooth (Fig. 8.4).

Having selected the appropriate shade of glass ionomer cement, the material is mixed and placed in one increment and the matrix is applied. Once the material has set, the matrix is removed and the filling is immediately protected with a layer of light-cured bonding resin. This prevents both the filling drying out and moisture contamination of the newly set material (Fig. 8.5). At this stage gross excess can be removed with a sharp carving instrument and the margin again covered with a light-cured bonding resin.

(a)   (b)

Fig. 8.4   (a) Tin-coated cervical matrices. (b) A coated tin cervical matrix in use. It has been attached to an instrument with sticky wax so that it can be held in place easily.

Fig. 8.5   Restoration of root caries with glass ionomer cement.
(a) The root caries was assessed as active, but the small enamel lesion on the mesial surface was considered to be arrested. Cavity preparation will remove all soft dentine. Hard but stained dentine will be retained and the arrested enamel lesion will not be included in the preparation (see p. 140).
(b) Immediately after restoring with glass ionomer cement. The rubber dam has just been removed. Further finishing will be carried out at a subsequent visit when the glass ionomer cement has fully matured. (Reproduced by courtesy of Mr N. L. Fisher.)

(a)   (b)

When a resin-modified glass ionomer material is chosen, where the set is initiated by light curing, any matrix must allow transmission of light. A capsulated material is easy to handle because the material can be injected directly into the cavity and the matrix can be adapted. The manufacturer's instructions should be followed with respect to curing time and depth of cure. In deeper cavities incremental build-up will be required, with each increment being light cured before the next is added. There is discussion as to whether these materials require protection to preserve water balance once the matrix is removed. The current consensus is that it would be wise to protect them with a layer of light-cured bonding resin.

Finishing

A high polish is particularly important on smooth surface restorations because plaque retention on the surface and around the margins can encourage further caries or gingival inflammation. In addition, the tongue and lips are sensitive to rough surfaces, particularly on the anterior teeth.

Composite restorations can be finished as soon as they have polymerized. Ledges can be removed with a fine flame-shaped 12-bladed tungsten carbide bur in the airotor handpiece, or alternatively diamond composite finishing burs can be used at high or low speed. Great care must be taken not to damage the tooth tissue around the filling. A series of composite finishing discs can then be used, and it is important to complete the process with the very finest of these to ensure that the filling is as smooth as possible.

Auto-cure glass ionomer cement restorations should not finally be finished for 24 hours (Fig. 8.5(b)). However, resin-modified light-cured materials have the advantage that they can be finished immediately. If care has been taken with the use of the matrix, minimal finishing is required. Multibladed tungsten carbide or diamond burs can be used at low speed to remove any ledges and the restoration finally smoothed with discs. The filling should be protected with a light-cured bonding resin.

It is difficult to avoid some minor trauma to the gingival margin while placing and finishing a cervical restoration. At a subsequent visit it is important to check that the gingival margin is healthy and that there are no areas of plaque retention.

EROSION—ABRASION LESIONS

These occur predominantly on the buccal and labial surfaces of teeth but may also occur lingually (Fig. 8.6). They are usually seen in one of two forms: a sharply outlined V-shaped notch (Fig. 1.36(b), p. 20) or a saucer-shaped lesion with rounded margins (Figs. 1.36(a) and 8.6). The V-shaped notches occur at the level of the cement–enamel junction and appear to be more common when there has been a degree of gingival recession. It is assumed that the defect starts primarily in the dentine, but enamel is also lost. Saucer-shaped defects occur anywhere on the buccal or labial surface but mostly on the necks of the teeth. They have a variety of shapes, and one common and unexplained variation is a groove running vertically up the buccal surface of the tooth (Fig. 8.7).

The aetiology of the lesions is unclear, although it has been assumed that vigorous tooth-brushing may be relevant. The extent to which this is important has not been established, and it is likely that chemical erosion also plays an important role. With this lack of understanding of aetiology it is difficult to prescribe logical treatment. If the aetiology is primarily chemical erosion, the wisdom of restoring the lesion at all must be questioned. The restoration will not prevent further erosion occurring around the margins. Indeed, the progress of the lesion may be accelerated as a result

Fig. 8.6 A sharply outlined V-shaped notch in the buccal surface of this extracted lower canine tooth. There is also a similar lingual defect but the aetiology of this is not clear. However, it seems likely that both lesions have some common aetiology and therefore incorrect tooth-brushing alone is unlikely to be the cause.

Fig. 8.7 Two study casts from the same patient taken three years apart. The upper cast shows defects starting on the lateral incisor and at the necks of the canine and first premolar teeth. In the lower cast these defects are all much deeper and better defined. The aetiology is unknown.

of chemical action in the deep narrow fissures around the restoration (Fig. 8.8(a)). Thus an unrestored wide shallow lesion may be less likely to progress. If the aetiology is not understood, prevention is likely to be ineffective and so the prognosis of many restorations placed in cervical erosion-abrasion lesions is poor.

For these reasons, a carefully considered decision must be made as to whether or not to restore a cervical erosion-abrasion lesion. There are three main reasons for placing a restoration:

- The area is sensitive and the sensitivity cannot be controlled by other means.

- The patient is concerned about the appearance of the lesion or has practical problems, such as food catching in the defect.

- The lesion is continuing to progress, and in particular is deepening, prejudicing the strength of the tooth and/or pulp vitality.

Sensitivity is surprisingly uncommon with the deeper lesions, presumably because of the defence reactions of the pulp–dentine complex, tubular sclerosis within the dentine, and reparative dentine at the pulpal surface. Early shallower cavities are often more sensitive and yet are not sufficiently deep to restore. In any case restorations do not reliably reduce sensitivity in these cases. Management should be aimed at encouraging more rapid deposition of reparative dentine and coagulation of the ends of the dentinal processes. This is achieved (sometimes only slowly) by the application of desensitizing toothpastes or varnishes (which contain fluoride) and by fluoride mouthrinses.

In the absence of a good reason for restoring the tooth, it is better to leave the lesion alone and continue to monitor it, intervening when one of the conditions above begins to apply. Intervention that is too early is likely to lead to repeated replacement restorations with a reduction rather than an improvement in the long-term prognosis of the tooth.

Choice of restorative material for abrasion—erosion lesions

The choice of material will depend on the known or assumed aetiology. If abrasion (physical wear) is regarded as the most important cause of the lesion, the restorative material must be capable of withstanding abrasive forces. Anterior composite materials are poor in this respect, and although composites have improved, they are not as good as amalgam, gold, or porcelain. However, these last three materials are not adhesive and therefore further preparation is required to make the cavity retentive. This is potentially very destructive and for this reason these materials have been almost entirely superseded by composite and glass ionomer cement. There has been a resurgence of interest in porcelain inlays, which undoubtedly have a very high abrasion resistance. It is possible to acid etch the fitting surface of the porcelain in the laboratory and then cement the restoration with composite resin cement. This may avoid the need for a retentive cavity preparation. However, such restorations have yet to be evaluated clinically and must be regarded as experimental at the moment (see Chapters 9 and 10).

At present, the most cost-effective solution is to use composite, and to replace the surface layer from time to time as necessary. In contrast with restorations involving the occlusal surface, wear does not potentially alter the occlusion and so this, 'wear and repair' approach is acceptable.

If the aetiology is thought to be primarily erosion and it is decided that a restoration is necessary, glass ionomer cement and composite restorations are the materials of choice. Most of these lesions have no enamel at the gingival margin and therefore layered restorations with both glass ionomer and composite are used.

(a)

(b)

(c)

Fig. 8.8 (a) A number of restorations presumably placed to treat erosion-abrasion cervical lesions. They have been unsuccessful in preventing further tooth wear around the restorations.
(b) Cervical notch-shaped lesions.
(c) The lesions were restored with the layered technique using glass ionomer cement and composite and this photograph was taken three years after the restorations were placed. No further wear has occurred and so it is likely that the aetiology (which was unknown) is no longer present.

Fig. 8.9 (a) Enamel hypoplasia on the buccal surface of the upper central incisor teeth.
(b) Shallow saucer-shaped cavities being prepared within the enamel using a diamond bur.
(c) Acid-etching gel being applied with a syringe.
(d) The etched surface being coated with bonding resin.
(e) Composite being applied from a capsule in a dispensing gun.
(f) A titanium nitride instrument being used to shape the composite.
(g) The composite being light cured.
(h) An orange protective shield in place to protect the eyes of the operator and dental nurse.
(i) A fine composite finishing diamond being used to shape the restoration.
(j) A finishing disc mounted on a plastic stub being used in the handpiece.
(k) The completed restoration.

Cavity preparation, lining, and filling

Most erosion-abrasion lesions do not require cavity preparation because tooth wear has produced a shape which can be filled with an adhesive material without further destruction of the tooth. The V-shaped groove is a good example of this (Fig. 8.8(b) and (c)). Any carious dentine within the lesion should be excavated or removed with a round bur at low speed.

Deep sensitive erosion-abrasion lesions may need a therapeutic lining containing calcium hydroxide. Where glass ionomer cement is to be used and no cavity preparation has been necessary, the polyacrylic acid conditioning solution supplied by the manufacturer should be used. This removes pellicle and facilitates the adhesion of the material. It is applied to the cavity on a small pledget of cotton wool and washed off after 10 seconds.

Matrices and filling techniques are the same as those described for the restoration of carious cavities.

ENAMEL HYPOPLASIA

In contrast with caries and erosion-abrasion lesions, enamel hypoplasia does not progress. Therefore it is not necessary to restore the tooth in order to treat a disease process, but fillings are sometimes required to improve appearance. For this reason these teeth are usually restored in young patients, and the type of restoration will depend on the extent of the lesion. When the entire surface of several teeth is affected, as in fluorosis, one of the veneering techniques (see Chapter 9) or a crown is used. However, with localized lesions, a more conservative approach is to prepare a shallow cavity and place a composite restoration (Fig. 8.9).

It is usually possible to do this without a local anaesthetic. If the base of the cavity is left in the enamel, then the entire surface can be etched before placing a composite and no lining is needed. It is only necessary to remove the whole thickness of the enamel if the tooth is discoloured to such a degree that it will not be masked by a relatively thin layer of composite. If dentine is exposed, it must be covered with calcium hydroxide or glass ionomer cement before the enamel is acid etched.

Since appearance is of prime importance, a microfine composite should be chosen. Application of the matrix and filling techniques are as described previously.

SUMMARY OF THE CHOICE OF RESTORATIVE MATERIALS FOR SMOOTH SURFACE LESIONS

With the developments in adhesive restorative materials, amalgam now has virtually no place in the restoration of the initial smooth surface lesions described in this chapter. The wear resistance and appearance of composite, together with the adhesive and cariostatic properties of glass ionomer cement, make the layered restoration the first choice in many cavities of large or moderate size involving enamel. With root caries, glass ionomer cement (or cermet) alone is the preferred choice. Amalgam is to be considered when the new restoration is to replace a failed amalgam and the tooth has already been prepared with undercuts. However, even here an adhesive restoration is often better.

FURTHER READING

Mount, G. J. (1994). *An atlas of glass ionomer cements. A clinician's guide* (2nd edn). Martin Dunitz, London.

9 Treatment of approximal caries, trauma, developmental disorders, and discoloration in anterior teeth

CONDITIONS AFFECTING ANTERIOR TEETH WHICH MAY NEED RESTORATIONS

Smooth surface caries, which affects the labial surfaces of anterior teeth but rarely the palatal or lingual surfaces, was dealt with in Chapter 8.

The other conditions affecting anterior teeth are as follows:

- approximal caries
- approximal caries which also involves the incisal edge
- trauma
- developmental disorders
- discoloured teeth
- tooth wear.

Approximal caries

Enamel caries starts on the approximal surface of anterior teeth just gingival to the contact area. It is less common than pit and fissure caries or caries in the approximal surfaces of posterior teeth. This is because the anterior teeth are more accessible for cleaning and the contact area is narrower. Caries may be more likely to occur when the teeth are crowded and overlapping, because this increases the difficulty in cleaning between them.

It is difficult to diagnosis early enamel caries at the white spot lesion stage, and so when a patient presents with established caries into dentine in one or more anterior teeth it is possible that the other contact areas have early enamel lesions. For this reason preventive treatment is important, including suitable dietary advice, the use of fluoride supplements (toothpaste, rinses, varnishes) and teaching the patient to use dental floss interproximally.

Dentine caries can usually be seen by transilluminating the tooth, either with light reflected from the mouth mirror (Fig. 9.1) or by a fibre-optic light (Fig. 1.22). Transillumination is more effective with anterior than posterior teeth because they are thinner. If dentine caries is visible, then it is usually too late for a 'prevent and observe' approach; a restoration is needed.

Fig. 9.1 Caries in dentine on the mesial aspect of an upper lateral incisor. The lesion is viewed in the dental mirror and is more obvious because light is passing *through* the tooth (transillumination).

Approximal caries which also involves the incisal edge

A neglected carious lesion, or secondary caries around an approximal restoration, may undermine the enamel of the incisal edge to the point where the corner of the incisor breaks away under occlusal forces. Dentine caries balloons out in all directions from its approximal origin, and by the time that it undermines incisal enamel it is often close to, or already affecting, the pulp. The diagnosis of the caries is straightforward, but a vitality test and periapical radiograph are required to assess any pulpal involvement and/or spread of infection into the periapical tissues.

Trauma

Accidental damage to teeth has one of the following effects (see Chapter 1):

- fracture of the incisal edge involving enamel only

- fracture involving enamel and dentine

- fracture involving enamel, dentine, and pulp

- root fracture

- cracks in the crown of the tooth without loss of enamel

- no visible damage but damage to the pulp or its blood supply, leading in the long term to pulp necrosis

- partial or complete luxation of the tooth.

The restoration of enamel and dentine fractures will be dealt with here; the other conditions are beyond the scope of this book. A broken incisal corner involving the incisal edge and parts of the approximal surfaces is treated rather similarly to approximal caries which involves the incisal edge.

Developmental disorders

In Chapter 8 small areas of enamel hypoplasia were considered, and the treatment technique described involved preparation of the tooth and the insertion of a shallow restoration. In this chapter, larger areas of hypoplasia or discoloration will be discussed. The techniques described are also suitable for other malformations including diminutive or peg-shaped teeth.

Discoloured teeth

Several developmental disorders result in discoloured teeth. However, a common cause of a single discoloured tooth is pulp necrosis, where the breakdown products of haemoglobin discolour the dentine. A bleaching technique to improve the appearance of such teeth will be described in this chapter.

Tooth wear

Smooth surface tooth wear was dealt with in Chapter 8 (p. 144). Tooth wear involving the incisal edges will be discussed here. With modern diets, teeth do not wear appreciably at their approximal surfaces, although this did happen with primitive man.

TREATMENT OPTIONS

Composite resin materials came into general use in the late 1960s and early 1970s. This produced a revolution in the restoration of anterior teeth, allowing procedures to be undertaken, using the acid-etch retention technique, that were impossible with any previous material. Today, with the added versatility of light-curing materials, many anterior teeth which would previously have been treated by crowns or extractions can be restored simply.

Uses and limitations of anterior composite materials

Provided that the occlusion is favourable, virtually the entire crown of an anterior tooth can be built up with composite, at least as a short-term restoration. This means that the majority of teeth with approximal caries, caries or trauma affecting the incisal edge, and many of the developmental disorders can be treated with composite alone. Tooth wear affecting the incisal edges is less successfully treated with composite since it tends to wear away quickly or break off. If it remains in place, its abrasiveness may increase the rate of wear of the natural opposing teeth.

Composite is limited in its use by the fact that it has a relatively low abrasion resistance, although composites vary in this respect, and also it sometimes becomes stained or develops a rough surface. Generally speaking, composites with a higher proportion of resin are prone to staining and those with a higher proportion of coarser particle size filler become rough as the surface wears down. These rough surfaces accumulate both plaque and extrinsic stain. If the occlusion is unfavourable, composite in contact with the opposing teeth will tend to break or lose retention.

Composite materials for anterior teeth are available in a variety of shades and in more opaque or more translucent versions. With large restorations it may well be necessary to use more than one shade to produce gradual colour changes across the surface of a tooth to match adjacent teeth.

Retention of composite to dentine

Anterior composite material should *always* be retained to the enamel by the acid-etch technique, even if the cavity is naturally undercut. This increases the marginal seal and reduces staining at the margins. However, composite is not retentive to dentine. In cavities, where the entire periphery is enamel, this does not matter because retention to enamel is sufficient, but in larger cavities where part of the border is apical to the cement-enamel junction and therefore has no enamel, retention to dentine is necessary. This is achieved in one of two ways:

• by an intermediate layer of glass ionomer cement

• by means of a dentine bonding agent.

The traditional method of retention is by means of retentive grooves and/or pins, and these have served for many years. Many dentists routinely used retentive grooves in dentine and a pin to support and retain composite replacing a broken incisal corner. However, even gold-plated pins may produce some discoloration in the composite, and their insertion carries some risk to the pulp. The use of glass ionomer cements or dentine bonding agents has now made these methods unnecessary.

Dentine bonding agents have been available for several years but are still being evaluated. Although the clinical results and laboratory tests for the early materials showed them to be effective in retaining composite to dentine surfaces, it became apparent that they were hydrolysing in the long term and reducing the durability of the bond. In addition, polymerization shrinkage of the composite may cause high stress at the bond.

Another problem with several of the dentine bonding systems which have been developed over the last few years (and in many cases these have disappeared from the market) was the complexity of the systems, with several bottles of liquid to be applied for different times. Many dentists found this too confusing and time-consuming to bother with. The newer dentine bonding agents are simpler to use, but do not yet have long-term clinical trial results to support their application. Yet another problem in using dentine bonding agents is that with large restorations it is necessary to use incremental packing, which is fiddly and time-consuming.

In contrast, glass ionomer cements are retentive to dentine, release fluoride, and have less polymerization contraction so that they can be used in bulk to replace all the dentine, leaving space for one increment of composite to replace the enamel. Glass ionomer cements are now available both in their original auto-curing form and as resin-modified glass ionomer cements (see Chapter 3, p. 56).

This is a developing field, and clinical research in the next few years is bound to influence clinical practice. At present, with large restorations where additional retention to dentine is needed for composite, the preferred approach is the glass ionomer cement–composite layered restoration.

Porcelain veneers

Porcelain veneers are cemented with composite resin to cover all or part of the labial surface of an anterior tooth. Porcelain has been used for crowns for over a century and is a very satisfactory restorative dental material in that it maintains its colour and surface gloss and is compatible with soft tissues.

Indications for porcelain veneers are where one or a number of anterior teeth are discoloured or misshapen in such a way that it is necessary to cover the entire labial surface to disguise the problem and yet the other surfaces are sound. The advantage of porcelain over a composite veneer is that it is more durable in terms of colour and surface gloss, although it is more likely to fracture. The advantage of a porcelain veneer over a crown is that the tooth preparation is more conservative and also, because the palatal surfaces of upper incisor teeth are not prepared, the occlusion is not affected. However, some reduction of the labial surface is usually necessary and so the procedure is not reversible. The restorations are time-consuming and involve laboratory costs which are often as high per tooth as the cost of a crown. If the tooth being covered is very darkly stained, the thin veneer does not sufficiently disguise the colour and so it has to be made more opaque. For these reasons porcelain veneers have by no means replaced crowns and are unlikely to do so. However, they form a useful addition to the operative dentist's techniques. Brief details of the technique for making porcelain veneers are given in Chapter 10 (p. 174).

Other materials and forms of treatment

The other two tooth-coloured materials which have been used to restore anterior teeth in the past are silicate cement and acrylic resin (poly (methyl methacrylate)). Neither of these materials are used now for permanent restorations, but many patients still have restorations in one or other of them. Silicate has the advantage of leaching fluoride and so is similar to glass ionomer cement in producing caries resistance. Its main disadvantages were its poor strength, so that it could not be used for incisal edge restorations, its poor solubility, so that the surface became progressively lost in many cases, and its low pH before it set, so that careful precautions had to be taken to avoid pulpal damage.

Acrylic used as a direct filling material has a very high coefficient of thermal expansion and so expanded and contracted more than the adjacent tooth tissue, producing rapid marginal leakage. It did not prevent caries, and therefore secondary caries was common. It can readily be identified by its distinctive smell when it is cut in the mouth.

EXAMPLES OF ANTERIOR RESTORATIONS

To illustrate the principles of restoring anterior teeth a number of examples will be described which have wide application in similar situations. There is considerable variety in the design of anterior restorations, and so the concept of an 'ideal' cavity preparation is even less true for anterior teeth than it is for posterior teeth. The approach must always be one of 'problem solving', bearing in mind the basic principles described earlier:

* gain access (if necessary)

* remove caries (if any)

* design the restoration, including its retention, for the restorative material chosen

* complete the preparation

* place the restoration

* finish and monitor.

Restoration of approximal caries in an anterior tooth

Isolation

Many approximal cavities in anterior teeth are close to the gingival margin. This is because caries develops just apical to the contact area and, unless there has been gingival recession, the gingival papilla reaches almost to the contact point. For this reason it is often necessary to retract the gingival papilla in order to avoid the restoration becoming contaminated by blood or gingival exudate. Therefore rubber dam should be used in most cases, and a wedge or a floss ligature is a convenient way to retract the rubber and the underlying gingival papilla (see p. 85).

Access to the caries

In most cases, access is through the palatal or lingual surface. When the teeth are in good alignment and the thickness of enamel overlying the caries is roughly similar labially and lingually, it is better to leave the sound labial enamel because it will maintain its appearance better than the restoration. In addition, if access is gained from the labial side, leaving only a thin layer of enamel palatally, there is a risk that the palatal enamel may fracture if this area is subject to occlusal forces.

Exceptions to this are where the teeth are overlapping and the caries is much closer to the labial than the palatal or lingual side (Fig. 9.2). A typical approximal lesion in well-aligned teeth is shown in Figs. 9.3(a) and 9.3(b) and the access cavity is shown in Fig. 9.3(c). Access is gained by a small round diamond or tungsten carbide bur using the airotor, and the same instrument is used to remove carious enamel (Fig. 9.3(d)).

Removing the caries

Dentine caries is removed at low speed with a round steel bur (Fig. 9.3(e)). In this situation caries in dentine is almost hemispherical, in outline. The enamel-dentine junction is cleared first, and then residual caries is removed from the pulpal aspect of

(b)

Fig. 9.2 (a) Overlapping incisor teeth with caries in the mesial surface of the lateral incisor. Access from the lingual side would be very difficult.
(b) Access has been gained from the buccal surface.

Fig. 9.3 (a), (b) A typical approximal lesion in the distal surface of the central incisor in well-aligned teeth.

(c) Access has been gained through the palatal enamel.

(d) The carious enamel has now been removed but there is still caries at the enamel-dentine junction and over the pulp.

(e) A small round steel bur being used at low speed to remove dentine caries.

(f) The cavity is now caries-free.

(g) A glass ionomer cement lining has been placed. Note how well this matches the colour and translucency of natural dentine. This produces a better appearance through thin remaining buccal enamel than opaque lining materials.

(h) Acid-etching gel in place. The matrix strip and wedge are to protect the lateral incisor from being etched as well.

(i) The bonding resin has been applied.

(j) A suitably shaped finishing diamond is used to shape the palatal surface and remove any excess composite.

(k) The final finishing of the cervical margin is carried out with an abrasive strip.

(l) The finished restoration.

the cavity until either it is all removed or a decision is made to leave firm stained dentine close to the pulp. In larger lesions caries spreading along the enamel-dentine junction leads to decalcified enamel on the inner aspect, although the outer surface is sound. Although this enamel is thin and unsupported by dentine, if it is on the labial surface, it is well worth keeping for aesthetic reasons. It also increases retention of the restoration when it is acid etched on its inner aspect. A caries-free cavity is shown in Fig. 9.3(f).

Designing the cavity and producing retention

Often little more preparation is necessary at this stage. Many small and moderate-sized lesions are naturally undercut. However, sufficient retention for composite is achieved by acid etching enamel whether or not undercuts are present, and so it is not necessary to produce an undercut cavity deliberately. Usually there is a sufficiently large area of enamel, often on the inner aspect, for acid-etch retention. In the absence of this, some operators cut retentive grooves in the dentine cervically and occlusally with a small round bur at low speed, or bevel the outer aspect of the preparation to increase the enamel surface area for etching.

If there is no enamel left at the cervical part of the cavity, glass ionomer cement should be used to increase retention here.

The main other consideration in designing the the cavity is to remove vulnerable enamel which has been thinned out and makes contact with the opposing teeth in the occlusion. 'Unsupported' enamel which does not contact opposing teeth in occlusal movements should be left.

Lining

Approximal carious lesions in anterior teeth are not usually restored until caries is established in dentine. The pulp horn is often close to the base of the caries and a calcium hydroxide or glass ionomer cement lining is almost always required in these cavities. It is applied very carefully on a ball-ended applicator, or alternatively on the back of a suitably sized and shaped excavator (Fig. 9.3(g)).

With deeper cavities and where there is no enamel cervically, glass ionomer cement can be used both to increase retention and to act as a secondary lining over the calcium hydroxide. In this case the glass ionomer cement is placed both in the base of the cavity and on the dentine of the cervical wall. The cement is applied on a ball-ended applicator.

Etching

Access to the enamel surfaces to be etched, including the inner aspects of the enamel, is often difficult if a brush or pledget of cotton wool is used. If these are used to apply etching fluid or gel, the etching may be incomplete or large areas of enamel may become etched unnecessarily. One solution to this problem is to use brightly coloured, and therefore clearly visible, etching gel applied through a blunt needle or a specially produced disposable nozzle from a syringe. With this technique the gel can be deposited only where it is wanted, without excess (Fig. 9.3(h)). The enamel of the adjacent tooth should be protected with a mylar matrix strip.

Bonding

The unfilled bonding resin is painted onto the etched area, taking care to produce a thin even layer (Fig. 9.3(i)) and the bonding resin is light cured.

Matrixing and packing

A thin flexible transparent matrix strip, which may be straight or curved, is used. It should be compatible with the resin being used, and polyester or mylar strips are preferred. The older type of cellulose acetate strip is not suitable, partly because it reacts with some types of resin and also because the strips are too thick and tear readily.

The strip should be well adapted to the cervical margin of the cavity and a wedge should be used to adapt the matrix in this area. It is particularly important to avoid creating a ledge cervically since it is difficult to remove an excess from this area. If access has been from the palatal or lingual side, one end of the matrix strip is pulled round to the labial side and held with a finger. The composite is inserted from the palatal or lingual side, the matrix is pulled round, and the composite is light cured from the palatal or lingual side through the matrix and from the labial side through the thin enamel.

Finishing

If the matrix has been adequate, it should not be necessary to finish the labial or cervical margins. A small cervical ledge can be removed, with difficulty, with a flexible impregnated strip. If there is a large cervical ledge, the filling should usually be replaced. Any excess on the palatal or lingual aspect can be trimmed with one of the following:

- a composite finishing diamond used at high or low speed (Fig. 9.3(j))

- a white stone used at low speed

- a multibladed tungsten carbide finishing bur in the airotor.

A final finish is given with a succession of abrasive discs, if access is sufficient for them, or mounted pumice-impregnated points or abrasive strips (Figs. 9.3(k) and 9.3(l)).

Composite restorations involving the incisal edge

Cavity preparation

Once the cavity includes the incisal edge, whether it is the result of caries, a previous failed restoration, or trauma, there is no difficulty in gaining access to the lesion and removing any caries that is present (Fig. 9.4(a)). The problem with the design of these restorations is to achieve adequate retention. For these reasons *all* the remaining labial enamel should be preserved (Fig. 9.4(b)). Unsupported enamel at the incisal edge which is in direct contact with the opposing teeth may need to be removed, but even this will usually be kept.

When the lesion is deep, a calcium hydroxide lining is placed immediately over the pulp. A glass ionomer cement is placed over this and extended onto the dentine, forming the cervical margin of the cavity. An auto-curing or resin-modified material maybe chosen, but the latter has the advantage that free radicals in the resin component will link chemically with the composite resin.

When the lesion is a result of trauma, the dentine and enamel surfaces may be fractured flush with each other and the dentine is not hollowed out as it is with caries. This means that there is not a large internal surface of enamel available for etching, and so with these lesions it is more usual to bevel the external surfaces of the enamel to increase the surface area for retention. The dentine is protected with a lining material in the usual way before etching the enamel and applying the bonding resin.

(a) **(b)** **(c)**

(d) **(e)** **(f)**

(g) **(h)**

Fig. 9.4 (a) A lesion involving the incisal edge.
(b) The cavity has been prepared by bevelling
the margins. A calcium hydroxide based lining
material has been applied and the enamel
etched.
(c) The matrix strip in place and the first
increment of composite being applied.
(d) The matrix is adapted with an instrument
and the first increment cured.
(e) Further increments are added, holding the
matrix with instruments or fingers but ensuring
that it is tightly adapted to the cervical margin
to reduce excess here. Incisal excess can easily
be removed with burs later.
(f) Final finishing of the cervical margin with an
abrasive strip.
(g), (h) The completed restoration. (This
restoration was carried out by an undergraduate
dental student.)

Matrixing, packing, and finishing

It is possible to trim a cellulose acetate crown form (used to make temporary crowns)
to act as a matrix for these restorations, attempting to adapt the margins of the
matrix around the entire periphery of the cavity. However, this technique is time-
consuming and elaborate and despite all this care it is not possible to adapt all the
margins perfectly and insert exactly the right amount of composite; therefore there
is always an excess of material to be removed. In addition cellulose acetate is not a
good matrix material for composite, as explained on p. 155. A simpler technique,
which fulfils the important requirements, is to use a simple Mylar strip matrix
properly adapted and wedged to the cervical margin interproximally but allowing an
excess of material to protrude incisally where it is easy to remove (Figs. 9.4(c),
9.4(d), and 9.4(e)).

Since these restorations are complex to contour and to achieve a realistic
appearance, the composite material is sometimes built up in increments, with each
increment being light cured before the next is added. Opaque 'dentine' shades are
used first and then a more translucent shade is used for the incisal edge. Either an
excess is left incisally, which is trimmed away later, or the last increments are placed
without the matrix strip and adapted to shape free-hand before curing.

There is usually good access for finishing these restorations with a succession of
composite finishing abrasive discs and strips (Figs. 9.4(f), 9.4(g), and 9.4(h)).

Veneering techniques for hypoplastic and discoloured teeth

When the aesthetic problem is such that a restoration inserted into part of the labial surface (see Chapter 8, p. 146) will not suffice, there is a choice of three restorative techniques:

- a composite veneer
- a porcelain veneer
- a crown.

Composite veneers

A major advantage of this technique is that it can be used without any preparation of the enamel, other than acid etching, so that it is an almost entirely reversible procedure. It is atraumatic and there is no need for a local anaesthetic or for the enamel to be cut; therefore it can be undertaken on very young or very nervous patients without great difficulty.

If the tooth is not discoloured at the gingival margin, the composite can be tapered down to a knife-edge finish cervically leaving a margin that is easy to clean.

A variety of complicated techniques for applying the matrix have been advocated for these restorations, but by far the simplest technique is to build up light-cured composite material free-hand on the surface of the tooth, altering the shade as necessary cervically and incisally. Very thin Teflon-coated flat plastic instruments have been designed for this. It is helpful to use a matrix strip between the teeth to avoid the enamel bond or composite becoming attached to the adjacent tooth. However, that is all the matrix that is usually required.

It is often better to place these restorations without rubber dam. The gingival condition should be healthy before these restorations are placed, and there is no tooth preparation so that there is no risk of gingival bleeding or exudate. Placing the restorations without rubber dam enables the optimum appearance to be achieved and the restoration can be contoured to finish just supragingivally so that it can be cleaned.

Finishing is with abrasive discs and, if necessary, with strips interproximally (Fig. 9.5).

Fig. 9.5 (a) The upper left lateral incisor is peg-shaped and the central incisors are small and taper towards the incisal edge. The patient was unhappy about the appearance of the spaces.
(b) Acid-etching gel applied to the three incisors. (NB This photograph was taken in 1983 before rubber gloves were worn routinely.)
(c) A well-etched enamel surface.
(d), (e) The three composite veneers which have been present for two and a half years at the time that these photographs were taken. There has been some slight dulling of the surface but no discoloration and the appearance is very satisfactory.

(a)

(b)

(c)

(d)

(e)

With discoloured teeth it is usually necessary to remove some enamel, particularly at the cervical margin. A long tapered round-end diamond bur in the airotor is used for the preparation, which must be done with great care so that the enamel is not penetrated, otherwise acid etching will not be possible. The enamel may be less than 0.5 mm thick in the cervical region so that particular care is needed to avoid overcutting and exposing dentine.

For stained teeth there are opaque composite materials which disguise the stain but which leave a rather dead-looking appearance. A better appearance is usually achieved with a porcelain veneer or with a crown but at the cost of more extensive tooth preparation.

Porcelain veneers

In most cases tooth preparation is necessary for porcelain veneers because the veneer cannot be tapered off to a knife-edge cervically without becoming too fragile to handle prior to cementation. Adding a thickness of porcelain cervically without tooth preparation will leave a ledge and a consequent problem with plaque removal. The technique has some similarities to that for inlays in that an impression is taken and the restoration made in the laboratory. Therefore the technique is described and illustrated in Chapter 10 (p. 174)

BLEACHING DISCOLOURED ANTERIOR TEETH

In some cases it is possible to bleach discoloured anterior teeth rather than veneer or crown them (Fig. 9.6). This is most successful in the case of an individual tooth which is discoloured as a result of haemoglobin breakdown products arising from a necrotic pulp which was not removed promptly enough. Claims have been made for successful bleaching of vital teeth with tetracycline staining or other intrinsic stains, but the results are less predictable and when the stain is not uniform the result is likely to be disappointing.

An individual non-vital tooth discoloured by haemaglobin breakdown products must initially be root filled with an inert material which does not itself discolour the crown (e.g. laterally condensed gutta-percha points with a white sealing paste). The tooth to be bleached must be isolated with rubber dam. The filling is removed from the access cavity and the access cavity enlarged, removing as much stained dentine as possible without weakening the tooth too much. This leaves a thin uniform layer of dentine through which the bleaching agents can percolate.

The dentine surface is etched for one minute with 30–50 per cent phosphoric acid to remove the smear layer and thus improve its permeability. A pledget of cotton wool soaked in the bleaching solution is inserted into the access cavity. A strong light (e.g. a composite polymerizing light) or heat is applied to the tooth for two to three minutes to accelerate the bleaching process. After this time the pledget of cotton wool is removed, the bleaching solution is washed away, and the tooth is inspected. The process may be repeated a number of times until the colour is about right. It is good practice to overbleach the tooth slightly as very commonly some further discoloration of the tooth reappears over a period of weeks after the procedure.

A variety of bleaching solutions have been used. Thirty per cent (or 100 volume) hydrogen peroxide has been the most commonly used and works in most cases. It is sometimes mixed with sodium perborate powder to accelerate the release of oxygen.

Hydrogen peroxide at this concentration is a very irritant material and there is concern (but little evidence) that it may be carcinogenic. For this reason materials providing more than 0.1 per cent of hydrogen peroxide have been banned in the United Kingdom from use on the external surface of teeth by either dentists or in the

(a)

(b)

(c)

Fig. 9.6 (a) A very discoloured upper right central incisor.
(b) The same tooth after bleaching.
(c) The endodontic access cavity must be opened up and the root filling removed to the level of the gingival margin. This allows good access to the dentinal tubules over the entire labial surface and also produces a reasonably thin layer of dentine and enamel to be bleached. (Figs 9.5 (a) and 9.5(b) by courtesey of Miss K. Warren. Reproduced from *Restorative Dentistry* by permission of A. E. Morgan Publications Ltd.)

'home bleaching' systems which were available until 1993. The legal position with respect to the use of materials containing more than 0.1 per cent of hydrogen peroxide on the internal surfaces of teeth is not entirely clear, but if it is used it must only be applied with rubber dam and eye protection in place, and with careful protection of the patient's clothes in case the solution drips off the bottom of the rubber dam while it is being washed away. A layer of Vaseline may be applied to the gingivae before the dam is placed. Good aspiration and plenty of water when washing are necessary. Care must be taken to avoid bleaching solution being drawn around the gingival margin by capillary action and trapped there by the rubber dam.

If the colour of the tooth does not change enough, a mixture of sodium perborate and hydrogen peroxide can be sealed into the access cavity with cotton wool and a temporary zinc oxide and eugenol dressing. This dressing can be left in place for a week. Cases of external resorption have been reported following bleaching, but it is not always clear whether these are the result of the bleaching or of the trauma or other condition which resulted in the necrotic pulp in the first place.

Once the tooth is bleached the dentine is replaced by a glass ionomer cement restoration. This bonds to the remaining dentine and enamel and strengthens the tooth. The palatal access cavity is then finally restored with composite which is acid-etch retained to the enamel margins and the glass ionomer cement.

FURTHER READING

Jordon, R. (1986). *Esthetic composite bonding*. Blackwell, Oxford.
Fisher, N. L. and Radford, J. R. (1990) Internal bleaching of discoloured teeth. *Dent. Update* **17**, 110–14.

10 Cast metal and porcelain intracoronal restorations

PLASTIC COMPARED WITH RIGID RESTORATIONS

Most of the restorations described so far have been plastic in the sense that the restorative materials used (amalgam, composite, and glass ionomer cement) have been in a plastic mouldable state as they were being inserted into the cavity and subsequently set to become rigid. The restorations to be described in this chapter are all constructed outside the mouth from rigid materials and are then cemented into the prepared tooth, which clearly must not be undercut.

The lost wax process

The modern cast restoration owes its development to an American dentist, Dr William H. Taggart, who in 1907 described a technique to produce gold castings which fitted prepared teeth with precision. The technique he refined is known as the *lost wax process* and involves making a wax pattern of the restoration which is then invested in a freshly mixed refractory material contained in a metal casting ring. When the investment has set, the whole is heated to a high temperature, causing the wax to burn out, leaving a space. Molten metal or glass is forced into the mould to form a replica of the original wax pattern.

Direct and indirect techniques

These are two methods by which cast metal restorations can be made (Fig. 10.1). In the *direct* method the wax is inserted directly into the cavity and the pattern is carved in the mouth and then invested and cast. It is taken to the chairside after polishing but with the margins untouched. Final finishing of the margins is then carried out in the mouth. Where the restoration is simple this technique is quick, accurate and saves both time and expense. However, single cavities can be satisfactorily restored with plastic materials and so the direct cast restoration is used very little today because it requires two visits by the patient, and is therefore expensive in time, and the amount of tooth tissue which must be restored to produce a non-undercut but retentive preparation for a cast restoration is greater than for an equivalent plastic restoration. Despite these reservations, the direct method will be described because it illustrates the principles simply, and because it is sometimes indicated, it should still be part of the dentist's repertoire.

In the *indirect* method an impression of the cavity and the surrounding area is made in the mouth. From this impression a model of the tooth, a die, is constructed. The wax pattern is formed upon this die, invested, and cast. It is fitted and finished on the die in the laboratory. Thus, only minimal adjustment should be required at the chairside, as the majority of the work has been carried out on accurate models in the optimum conditions of the laboratory. This is the technique of choice for all complex restorations.

Direct Technique

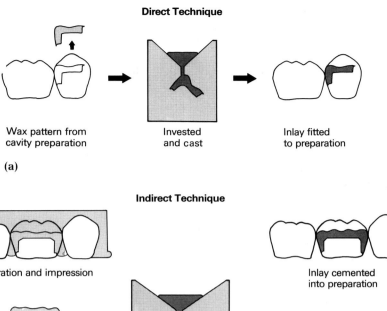

Fig. 10.1 Alternative methods for producing cast metal restorations.

Wax pattern from   Invested   Inlay fitted
cavity preparation   and cast   to preparation

(a)

Indirect Technique

Preparation and impression   Inlay cemented
into preparation

Wax pattern from model   Investment and casting   Inlay fitted to model

(b)

Intracoronal and extracoronal restorations

There is no clear dividing line between intracoronal and extracoronal restorations. A restoration contained within an occlusal cavity is clearly intracoronal, and a complete crown is clearly extracoronal; however, between these two extremes there are a number of restorations which are more difficult to categorize. A cast metal inlay which also covers the entire occlusal surface of a posterior tooth is partially intracoronal and partially extracoronal. Traditionally, extracoronal restorations have been considered as complete or partial crowns made of metal or porcelain; however, a composite labial veneer applied to the etched enamel surface must surely be regarded as an extracoronal restoration although it does not fit into the traditional definition.

The restorations to be described here are those which can reasonably be regarded as alternatives to the plastic restorations described earlier and are mostly intracoronal. Complete and partial crowns will not be described, as planning for these introduces another set of considerations beyond the scope of this book. Also, many additional clinical and laboratory techniques are necessary and as these are similar to those used in the construction of bridges it is more logical to consider crowns and bridges together. The restorations to be considered here are as follows:

- cast metal inlays produced by the direct method
- cast metal inlays and onlays produced by the indirect method
- porcelain inlays
- porcelain veneers.

MATERIALS
Cast metal

The traditional material for inlays is gold. Pure gold (24 carat, 100 per cent, or 1000 fine) is seldom if ever used as it is a very soft material. Other metals are added to improve the physical properties, and therefore the material used in a traditional 'gold' inlay is in fact a gold alloy. In some cases alloys containing 60 per cent or more of gold are still used and these can reasonably be described as **gold** alloys. However, the high cost of gold has stimulated development and improvements in other alloys and a vast choice is now available to the clinician and technician. Some alloys which are used for intracoronal restorations contain only 20 per cent or so of gold and so it is misleading to describe these as 'gold' alloys. Other alloys contain no gold at all but are based on a combination of other metals. This is why the term 'cast metal' has been used so far in this chapter.

Despite the improvements in low gold alloys, they remain more difficult to work with than the traditional high gold alloys. High gold alloys should still be used for inlays because the amount of metal used is small and therefore the added cost is relatively insignificant. A textbook on dental materials should be consulted for a detailed comparison of the properties of various types of casting alloys.

Porcelain

Porcelain inlays and veneers are made by one of two completely different techniques. In the first technique, the impression of the tooth is cast in a refractory material which can be heated to very high temperatures without damage. Porcelain powder is mixed to a paste with a liquid and placed into the inlay cavity or onto the labial surface of this refractory model and is then fired in a furnace until the particles of porcelain fuse together. The process is repeated a number of times until the restoration is built to the required contour and colour. The refractory model is then removed, usually by sand (or glass bead) blasting.

The second method is to cast an ingot of castable glass into a mould made by the lost wax technique. This glass restoration is then treated in a ceramming furnace which converts the material to a ceramic which is then surface stained and fired to change its appearance. Both techniques produce a ceramic restoration (commonly, but not really accurately, called porcelain) but the materials have rather different properties. Again, a textbook of dental materials should be consulted for the details of these differences.

ADVANTAGES AND DISADVANTAGES OF CAST METAL AND PORCELAIN RESTORATIONS
Strength

Cast metal is stronger in thin sections than amalgam, composite, or glass ionomer cement, and it has a greater ability to resist tensile forces. Thus, it is the material of choice to protect weakened cusps where a metal thickness of 1.0 mm or even less is sufficient compared with a minimum thickness of 3 mm for amalgam. Its strength in thin sections also makes it ideally suited for extracoronal veneer restorations such as onlays and complete and partial crowns. Preparations for cast metal restorations are usually finished with bevelled or chamfered margins to give a thin edge of metal.

In contrast, porcelain has high compressive strength but low tensile strength. This means that it is relatively brittle in thin sections, at least until it is bonded to the tooth and supported by it. Therefore porcelain restorations should not have bevelled margins, and a minimum thickness is necessary to avoid fracture of the restoration.

For a conventional porcelain crown this thickness is about 1.5 mm, but for porcelain veneers which are not subjected to occlusal forces 0.5 mm or less may be sufficient.

Abrasion resistance

Although amalgam is similar to enamel in resisting abrasion, both composite and glass ionomer tend to wear more rapidly than enamel, particularly on the occlusal surface. Cast metal and porcelain are at least as resistant to abrasion as enamel, and indeed there has been some concern that porcelain is more resistant so that if a porcelain restoration is opposed by a natural tooth, the natural tooth may wear down more rapidly. This will certainly happen if the glaze on the porcelain is inadequate or has been ground off. With an abrasion cavity at the neck of the tooth, composite or glass ionomer may be inadequate to resist further abrasion and porcelain or cast metal inlays are sometimes used to overcome this problem (Fig. 10.2).

Fig. 10.2 Porcelain inlays used to restore cervical lesions in all four teeth. These porcelain inlays were made by traditional techniques 25 years ago.

Appearance

At one time, when the choice of restorative material was amalgam, gold, or silicate, gold was frequently preferred for aesthetic reasons as it was more attractive than amalgam and did not deteriorate like silicate. Also, in many societies it was regarded as a status symbol to have gold visible in the front or to the side of the mouth. With the introduction of more reliable tooth-coloured restorative materials this fashion tended to die away and relatively few patients now ask for visible gold restorations.

Porcelain, in contrast can have a very natural appearance, and in some situations it is the material of choice for this reason. Its appearance, once established, is very durable compared with composite and glass ionomer which sometimes discolour or develop stained margins.

Versatility

Cast metal is a very versatile material. The indirect technique allows it to be shaped accurately in the laboratory to restore occlusal and axial contours and contact areas. Where cast restorations are placed in patients for whom partial dentures are to be made, it is possible to build appropriate guiding planes, rest seats, and reciprocal ledges into the cast restoration at the laboratory stage. If advantage is to be taken of this situation, it is absolutely essential that the partial denture be designed before the cast restoration is made. In addition, cast metal can be soldered and thus contact areas can be added at the fit stage. These alloys are almost unchallenged as the materials of choice for bridgework.

Cost

Cost is the major disadvantage of cast metal and porcelain restorations. The reason for the high cost is the amount of time that they take compared with plastic restorations. There is always a laboratory stage and so a minimum of two clinical appointments is necessary, the first to prepare the tooth and take an impression and the second to fit the restoration after it has been made in the laboratory. This extra time taken by the dentist and the technician means that these restorations are inevitably several times more expensive than the equivalent plastic restoration. This extra cost has been seen in the past as giving further status to the restorations, particularly gold inlays. It was assumed that because a gold inlay costs several times more than an amalgam restoration it must be several times better. This does not automatically follow. Certainly a gold inlay has some advantages over amalgam in that it does not corrode or discolour the tooth and it is stronger. However, in choosing between the materials a proper cost–effectiveness analysis is needed rather than looking at the cost alone or the effectiveness alone.

Using alloys with less gold (or in some cases none) reduces the cost of the material a little but does not save time, and so the overall cost is still high.

The cement lute

The weak link in any cemented restoration is the cement lute. The margin of even a well-fitting cast metal restoration is some micrometres away from the cavity wall (10–60 μm). Thus, the marginal seal of the restoration is entirely dependent upon the cement lute, whereas the seal of an amalgam restoration is good as corrosion products tend to block the initial microspace. Fortunately, glass ionomer cements are now available for luting and, because these materials contain available fluoride, cemented restorations may now have a better prognosis in a caries-prone mouth. However, this hypothesis has yet to be tested in clinical trials.

Indications

Bearing these points in mind, the following are the most common indications for each type of restoration although, of course, there will be many variations when the needs of individual patients have been taken into account.

Direct cast metal inlays

As will be seen later, the technique for direct cast metal inlays is such that they can only reasonably be made for very small cavities. This being so the strength of the cast metal has very little advantage and the cost of the procedure is very rarely justified. Only a small number of direct cast metal inlays are made, and these are usually indicated in conjunction with some other restoration; for example, a buccal inlay with a dimple on the surface to provide an undercut for the retentive clasp arm of a partial denture or as the minor retainer for a fixed, movable, or hybrid bridge (see textbooks on crowns and bridges).

Indirect cast metal inlays

The indirect technique allows a much greater range of preparation design and the most commonly made type of cast metal inlay is used to protect the cusps by covering the occlusal surface. These are called either inlays with cuspal protection or onlays. The second most common indication for indirect inlays is as part of a bridge or other appliance replacing missing teeth.

Porcelain inlays

Porcelain inlays were used occasionally in the past (Fig. 10.2) but with the introduction of composite materials they fell into disuse. However, a new generation of materials and techniques has been developed in the last few years and there has been a resurgence in interest in porcelain inlays. As yet, it is too early to say what their long-term clinical success is and therefore exactly when they should be prescribed.

However, porcelain inlays or onlays have the advantages that they are more natural in appearance than cast metal inlays and are more abrasion-resistant than composite. Therefore they may be appropriate in the occlusal surfaces of posterior teeth when large restorations are needed and appearance is important. They may be used in the buccal surfaces of visible anterior and posterior teeth when abrasion is a problem. They are not as strong as cast metal inlays but when they are bonded to the enamel surfaces of weakened cusps using the acid-etch technique, it is likely that they strengthen the tooth in much the same way as composite or glass ionomer–composite layered restorations. This means that full protection of the occlusal surface of the weakened cusp may not be necessary as it is with cast metal inlays.

Porcelain veneers

The general indications for veneering the labial surface of teeth were described in Chapter 9. When a veneer is indicated, the choice of material is between composite and porcelain. Composite has the advantage of being versatile and it can usually be placed without any tooth preparation. This means that the process is largely reversible. The margin can be feathered off at a sharp bevel, producing little change in the contour of the tooth at the cervical margin and interproximally. However, composite tends to wear and sometimes discolours. For these reasons porcelain is sometimes preferred and in most cases the tooth needs to be prepared to accommodate the porcelain veneer, particularly at the margins, since the veneer cannot be finished to such a fine bevel. This means that the process is not reversible. The cost is also high because the veneers have to be made individually in the laboratory and in many cases several teeth need to be treated. However, porcelain veneers may give a very durable and unchanging appearance, and although tooth preparation is necessary, they are more conservative of tooth tissue than a conventional complete crown.

PREPARATIONS AND CLINICAL TECHNIQUES

Direct cast metal inlay

Figure 10.3(a) shows the design features of a preparation for an inlay in the buccal surface of a premolar tooth. The important characteristic of the preparation is that it should not be undercut and yet be as retentive as possible. Theoretically, the angle between the walls of the cavity should be 7–10 degrees, but this is almost impossible to achieve clinically, and measurements of preparation tapers undertaken for large numbers of clinical preparations show an average taper of about 20 degrees. This is clinically acceptable, and in any case the actual angle is irrelevant as no attempt is made to measure it clinically. In examining an inlay cavity clinically, one eye should be closed to ensure a single line of vision and by adjusting this to the path of insertion of the inlay it should be just possible to see all the internal surfaces of the preparation. If the internal surfaces are clearly visible, then the preparation is over-tapered. However, if one wall always remains out of sight, even if the dentist moves his or her head around, the cavity is undercut. The walls should be smoothly finished so that the direct pattern can be withdrawn. A straight-cut tapered fissure bur used at high or low speed is suitable for finishing.

A ductile alloy should be used and the margin of the cavity bevelled as shown in Fig. 10.3(a) so that the inlay can be burnished to improve marginal adaptation. Bevels can be cut at high speed with multibladed tungsten carbide burs or at low speed with steel or tungsten carbide finishing burs or with green stones.

The cavity can now be lined with glass ionomer cement. In a very deep cavity a calcium-hydroxide-containing cement would be needed as sublining.

The direct pattern

In most cases inlay wax is used but occasionally it may be more practical to use an acrylic resin material which is specifically produced for the purpose, so that when it is heated in the investment it burns out completely leaving no residue.

Fig. 10.3.   (a) An ideal preparation for a direct gold inlay. The walls should be near parallel and the cavo-surface angle is bevelled.
(b) The prepared cavity is lubricated with liquid paraffin (or the patient's saliva).
(c) A stick of inlay wax is softened, rounded to a point, and plunged into the cavity.
(d) The wax is held in place with a finger until it cools, leaving a gross excess.
(e) The wax is carved.
(f) The sprue in place.
(g) The finished wax pattern withdrawn. Note the reproduction of the bevelled margin.

(a)

(b)

(c)

(d)

(e)

(f)

(g)

To make a direct wax pattern the prepared tooth surface is first lubricated with a thin smear of liquid paraffin or soap solution (Fig. 10.3(b)). A stick of inlay wax is formed into a softened cone by gently warming the end of a stick above a spirit or gas flame. It is important that the wax should not be overheated to the extent of melting until it drips. The end of the stick is moulded to a pointed form between finger and thumb. The softened cone of wax is pressed into the cavity and firm finger pressure is applied until the wax cools (Figs. 10.3(c) and 10.3 (d)).

Once hard, the wax is carved with warmed or sharp instruments as shown in Fig. 10.3(e), taking care to reproduce the cavo-surface bevel and the contour.

The surface of the wax can be smoothed by moistening a pledget of cotton wool with water and holding it with tweezers in the flame until the water is near boiling. This can be used to smooth out fine irregularities.

The next stage is to *sprue* the pattern. The sprue consists of a piece of straight round wire approximately 1 mm in diameter and 15 mm long. It is warmed, and after adding a small quantity of inlay wax it is inserted into the centre of the pattern and allowed to cool (Fig. 10.3(f)). It serves two purposes, first as a handle to withdraw the pattern and second to form a channel through which the molten metal will flow after the pattern is invested and the sprue withdrawn.

The wax pattern is withdrawn from the cavity by holding the sprue in the fingers (rather than tweezers) and the fit surface of the pattern is closely inspected (Fig. 10.3(g)). There should be a sharp reproduction of the detail of the internal surface of the cavity. If internal angles appear dull and rounded it is likely that the wax was not sufficiently hot when inserted and the pattern must be retaken.

An acrylic resin pattern or a pattern consisting of a combination of acrylic resin or wax is made when a larger direct pattern is needed. The acrylic is stronger than wax and can be manipulated without so much risk of breaking. An example of when the technique is useful is when an occlusal–proximal restoration is needed in a tooth which already carries the rest seat of a satisfactory partial denture. Imagine that the rest of the denture fits into a rest seat in an amalgam restoration which has now failed and must be replaced. If a new amalgam is placed, it will be very difficult to carve so that the denture rest is a good fit on the occlusal surface. To ensure this with a gold inlay made by the indirect method the denture will have to be taken from the patient for a while so that the inlay can be made to fit it in the laboratory. A direct inlay technique can solve this problem. An acrylic resin pattern is built up with small increments of the powder–liquid mix on a paint brush until the pattern is just short of the denture. The denture is then lubricated and inserted in the mouth and more resin allowed to flow between the rest and the pattern. When this is set, the denture can be removed and then the pattern removed and trimmed with burs. Adjustment to the axial or occlusal contours can be made with inlay wax if necessary.

A temporary filling will be needed to protect the exposed dentine until the inlay is cast. This may simply be one of the premixed temporary cement materials, but one of the temporary crown and bridge acrylics is preferable because this can be properly shaped and then, when the gold inlay is ready to cement the temporary inlay, can be removed in one piece.

The acrylic is mixed to a dough consistency, placed into the cavity, and contoured with a flat plastic instrument. When nearly set it is eased out, and then replaced and withdrawn a number of times until it is set. This prevents the temporary inlay from sticking in the cavity. The temporary inlay is then cemented with a temporary zinc oxide and eugenol luting cement.

Laboratory stages

The laboratory stages will vary depending on the material of the pattern and the casting metal which is to be used. Very briefly, the sprue and pattern are sealed onto a cone-shaped form; this is covered by a casting ring and investment material is poured into the other end of the ring and allowed to set. When it is set, the former is removed and the sprue withdrawn with pliers. The ring is then heated in a furnace until the wax melts and evaporates or the acrylic burns away and then molten metal is cast into the cone-shaped end of the ring and allowed to set. When still hot the ring is dropped into water and the investment cracks and can easily be removed. The sprue is then cut, usually leaving a short length as a handle to help when trying the inlay in the mouth. Small direct inlays are usually not polished until they are tried in the mouth.

A suitable textbook should be consulted for more details of the laboratory stages involved in casting metals.

Fig. 10.4 Direct gold inlay which has been in the mouth for more than 30 years. (Compare this with Fig. 6.5.)

Fig. 10.5 A direct gold inlay made by one of the authors over 30 years ago.

The second clinical visit

The temporary filling should be removed and the cavity cleaned and inspected for any remains of temporary filling material. For most small inlays it is advisable to use rubber dam so that if the inlay is dropped there is no risk of the patient inhaling or swallowing it.

Before the inlay is tried in the cavity its fitting surface should be inspected under magnification. Occasionally small blobs of gold are seen. These have been caused by trapped air bubbles at the investment stage. One or two of these can be removed from the gold with a sharp excavator, but if these defects are large or numerous, the wax pattern should be retaken.

The inlay is tried in. If it does not seat, the cavity should be inspected for remnants of temporary cement. An alternative explanation for the problem is that the cavity was undercut and the wax pattern has distorted. In this case, the cavity must be modified and the pattern retaken. Sometimes these undercuts, and subsequent distortion of the wax, cause the inlay to appear to seat but rock in the cavity. Again, this defect will require cavity modification and a new wax pattern. Finally, the bevels should be checked because a deficient bevel will also require a new wax pattern.

If the restoration fits, the margins are burnished with a hand-held burnisher, moving the instrument from inlay to tooth. An area of the margin which appears to be too thick can be reduced with a small round steel finishing bur or a white stone used at low speed. The instrument should be used with a light touch and rotate from gold to tooth so that it has the effect of working the gold down onto the tooth surface. Once the metal has been thinned it can be reburnished with a hand instrument.

The margins are now polished in the mouth as far as possible, using rubber pumice points and cups. Finally, the inlay is removed and the sprue is cut off with a cutting disc in the straight handpiece, holding the inlay in pliers. The remainder of the surface is polished using an abrasive rubber wheel.

The inlay is now cemented either with glass ionomer luting cement or with zinc phosphate cement mixed to a creamy consistency. The former is preferable as it is more adhesive to dentine and less of an irritant to the dental pulp. The cement is mixed according to the manufacturer's instructions. The mixed cement is applied to the fitting surface of the inlay and the restoration is seated into the cavity and pushed into position with a pear-shaped burnisher. When the cement is fully set an excavator or probe is used to remove the excess. The restoration may be polished finally with rubber pumice points and the margins revarnished.

Figure 10.4 shows a gold inlay which has been in place for more than 30 years. This was made by the direct method. Figure 10.5 shows an inlay made by one of the authors in his final qualifying practical examination more than 30 years before this picture was taken.

Indirect cast metal inlay

Preparation for an MOD inlay with cuspal protection

This is the most common type of inlay still made. The preparation follows the general principles of cavity preparation and design described in Chapter 3. These principles are applied in rather different ways to take account of the properties of the materials being used, but remain essentially the same as for plastic restorations:

- gain access to the caries or remove the old restoration
- remove caries
- put the handpiece down and think.

The decision to make an inlay should be reconsidered at this stage and if the decision is confirmed details of the design should be planned.

- prepare the cavity to be retentive and resistant
- prepare cuspal coverage
- check for undercuts
- prepare finishing lines
- line the cavity.

Retention for inlay cavities

The general principles of retention were described in Chapter 3. Retention is achieved by preparing opposing walls as near parallel to each other as is practical (see p. 60) but without undercuts. This allows a single path of insertion from an occlusal direction, and is most conveniently achieved by cutting the preparation with a straight-cut taper-fissure tungsten carbide bur in the airotor. To achieve near-parallel walls the bur should be realigned very slightly when transferring from the buccal to the lingual side of the cavity. Loss of retention in other directions is prevented by the presence of cusps and by occlusal locks in much the same way as amalgam restorations are retained.

Cuspal coverage

The important aspect of the design and the main reason for choosing this type of restoration is to prevent the weakened cusps from breaking under occlusal pressures. To do this, the weakened cusps are reduced in height in a direction parallel to the slope of the cusp. The amount of reduction will depend on the circumstances but should not be less than 0.5 mm. In some cases it will need to be more (up to 1.5 mm), particularly when the cusp being protected is in contact in lateral movements of the mandible (a functional cusp) and therefore is vulnerable to lateral forces. In addition, the metal may wear and become thinner over a period of years. A typical design is shown in Fig. 10.6.

Fig. 10.6 (a) A typical design for an MOD inlay with cuspal protection for one wall of the tooth. (b) A cross-sectional view. The reverse bevel (B) produces an acute metal margin.

Checking for undercuts

The cavity must be free from undercuts so that it is possible to see all the line angles and corners of the cavity at once. This can be checked by looking into the cavity, either directly or with a mirror (preferably one which is surface-reflecting) in the line of withdrawal of the inlay. Without the operator moving his or her head a probe is passed along all the line angles and into all the corners of the cavity. If the point of the probe is lost from view, it will have entered an undercut. It is undoubtedly easier to look for undercuts with one eye shut in order not to be misled by binocular vision. In the MOD cavity particular care should be taken to ensure that the boxes are not undercut with respect to one another. Any undercut must be eliminated, either by further preparation of the tooth or, if it is well supported by dentine, by blocking out with glass ionomer cement.

Finishing lines

Some form of bevel or chamfer is the finishing line of choice for intracoronal cast restorations. Their use gives a cavo-surface angle of approximately 135 degrees and a gold margin angle of 45 degrees. When the inlay is fitted, this thin gold margin can be burnished onto the enamel.

Any functional cusp can be finished with a chamfer finishing line, bringing the margin of the gold away from the area of occlusal stress. This is cut with a tungsten carbide chamfer finishing bur used in the airotor. On non-functional cusps a reverse bevel should be cut with the airotor using a tungsten carbide finishing bur (Fig. 10.6).

With large boxes, bevels should be placed along the axial walls of the box and at the cervical margin. This is difficult but can be achieved with care using a straight-cut tapered tungsten carbide bur in a 1:4 ratio speed increasing handpiece. This bevel must be large if it is to avoid creating undercuts beneath the maximum bulbosity of the tooth. Care should be taken to merge these bevels with the occlusal bevels. The cervical margin bevel can be cut with a pointed, flame-shaped composite finishing diamond (Figs. 10.7(a) and 10.7(b)).

Cavity lining

In a deep cavity a sublining of a proprietary cement containing calcium hydroxide should be used. A second lining material should then be placed to line out any undercuts, flatten the occlusal floor and pulpal walls, and provide thermal insulation for the pulp. Glass ionomer cement is the optimum material for this structural lining because it is adhesive to dentine. It is often easiest to place a small excess of the material and, once it has set, cut it back to achieve a smooth and precise lining; every wrinkle is a possible source of error, as it is reproduced in the impression, the die, the wax, and the metal. The pulpo-axial line angle should be bevelled. If it is left sharp it will be reproduced in the investment, a relatively weak material which may be fractured as the molten alloy pours over it during the casting procedure.

Impressions

An impression of the cavity and the full arch of teeth is taken in an elastomeric impression material (Fig. 10.7(c)). The dentist may choose to use one of three groups of these materials: the polysulphides, polyethers, or silicones. A textbook of dental materials should be consulted for the chemical composition of the materials and the manufacturer's instructions should be read concerning the handling of the chosen material.

An impression of the opposing arch is taken, usually in alginate. An important feature of this impression is that the occlusal surface of the teeth should be recorded without air bubbles so that the opposing models can be articulated accurately.

(a)

(b)

(c)

(d)

(e)

Fig. 10.7 (a) A failed MOD amalgam restoration in the second premolar tooth. The cusps are thin and weak and, in addition, the tooth is to be used as a partial denture abutment.
(b) The cavity prepared for an MOD inlay with cuspal coverage. A glass ionomer cement lining has been placed.
(c) The impression in light and heavy-bodied silicone rubber impression material.
(d) The wax pattern on a removable stone die.
(e) The finished restoration cemented.

An interocclusal record will not be needed where there are sufficient occluding teeth. However, if there is any doubt about the occlusion, a suitable interocclusal record is taken in the intercuspal position.

The special tray
A special tray is recommended with several, but not all, the elastomeric impression materials. The tray supports the material around the teeth; this means that less impression material is used and ensures a consistent thickness of material. This may be relevant to the dimensional stability of the material.

When required, a special tray is made of acrylic resin on a study model. The tray should cover all the teeth in the arch and is extended 2 mm beyond the gingival margins. The tray is spaced over the teeth by 1–3 mm but contacts three or four teeth around the arch so that it can be seated accurately without touching the prepared tooth.

The correct adhesive for the impression material should be painted on the inside of the tray and around the margins and allowed to dry before the impression is taken.

Isolating the tooth : gingival retraction
The elastomeric impression materials are hydrophobic and so the prepared tooth surface must be dry. The tooth is isolated with cotton-wool rolls and a saliva ejector is placed in the mouth.

Careful management of the gingival tissues is the key to taking good impressions, since any gingival exudate or bleeding will prevent the material from flowing over the prepared tooth surface. It is essential that the gingival tissues are healthy before the preparation is started. When the preparation margin extends to or beneath the gingival margin, it is necessary to retract the gingival margin before taking the impression so that an accurate impression of the margin can be recorded.

A suitable gingival retraction cord impregnated with styptic, such as aluminium chloride, or a vasoconstrictor, such as adrenalin, is chosen. The latter would not be used in patients with cardiovascular problems or those taking tricyclic antidepressants because the adrenalin is readily absorbed. The cord is gently pressed into the gingival crevice with a flat plastic instrument. It is left for a minute or two before the impression is taken.

Taking the impression
The impression materials are mixed throughly, usually in an automix gun system, according to the manufacturer's instructions. The retraction cord is removed and a low-viscosity impression material is syringed into the preparation and around the tooth. A heavier-viscosity material or putty mix (the putty materials obviate the need for a special tray) is placed in the impression tray and the tray is seated over the unset low-viscosity material. This helps to adapt it into all the areas of the preparation and into the gingival crevice. The impression is supported while it sets and is then removed from the mouth.

Examining the impression
The impression of the prepared tooth should be examined in detail to check that the entire margin is visible and that there are no voids caused by air entrapment. The detail of the occlusal surface of the entire impression should also be checked because voids caused by air bubbles will subsequently fill with plaster and prevent accurate occlusion of the models (Fig. 10.7(c)).

The temporary inlay

While the cast inlay is being constructed an accurate temporary restoration is needed for the following reasons:
- to protect the pulp

- to prevent ingrowth of gingival tissues
- to prevent alteration of occlusal and approximal contacts
- to prevent fracture of weakened cusps
- to restore appearance and comfort.

A durable inlay is required that can be cemented with a temporary luting material but is easily removed at a subsequent visit. One of the temporary crown and bridge materials is conveniently made into a temporary inlay.

The cavity is lightly lubricated with Vaseline and a matrix band is fitted to the tooth. The band is burnished to obtain accurate approximal contacts, and wedges are placed to ensure good cervical adaptation. The resin is mixed and when it has a putty consistency it is firmly placed into the band. Alternatively the inlay can be made free-hand, without a band, which will produce more excess resin but this can easily be removed by trimming out of the mouth.

As the resin sets it loses its plasticity and the temporary inlay can now be removed. It should be replaced gently and withdrawn a number of times until it has set. Excess resin is now trimmed off the inlay outside the mouth with a bur or stone in a laboratory handpiece. Finally, the inlay is inserted and the occlusion is checked with articulating paper and adjusted until it is correct in intercuspal position and in lateral excursions. The temporary inlay is finally smoothed with a rubber wheel before cementing it with a zinc oxide and eugenol temporary luting cement. Once the cement has set, excess is removed with a probe.

Laboratory stages

Again, the laboratory procedures will not be described in detail. Basically, the working impression is cast in a hard artificial stone incorporating tapered pins or other devices to allow the model of the prepared tooth to be sawn out of the rest of the model in such a way that it can be re-inserted in the same position. This is the die. The wax pattern is made on the lubricated die and, because the die can be removed from the master model, more accurate adaptation of proximal gingival margins, contact points, etc. is possible than with a direct wax pattern (Fig. 10.7(d)). The wax pattern is then sprued as before, but usually with wax or plastic rather than metal, and cast as described on p. 167. The sprue is removed and the inlay polished in the laboratory before returning to the surgery.

The occlusion is checked while the wax pattern is being made and during polishing by articulating the working model with the opposing model. This can be done by hand, but it is very much better to articulate the casts in a simple articulator. The advantage is that with hand-held models the majority of teeth will come together even if the wax pattern or inlay are proud. However, with articulated models a high contact on the pattern will keep the other teeth apart and the occlusal discrepancy will be more obvious.

The second clinical visit

Before the patient arrives, the fit of the casting on the die should be checked and the fit surface examined for small excesses that could prevent the restoration from seating.

Removing the temporary inlay

It is not convenient to use a rubber dam when fitting a cuspal coverage restoration because the occlusion must be checked carefully. However, a moist piece of sponge, a *butterfly sponge*, can be placed in the mouth to prevent the inlay being swallowed or inhaled. A scaler is used to remove the temporary inlay and all traces of temporary cement are gently removed with a probe.

Trying in the casting

Having checked that the butterfly sponge is protecting the pharynx, seat the casting and check the margins with a sharp probe for deficiencies or ledges. If the casting will not seat, look for causes in the following sequence:

- Debris or temporary cement still in the preparation.

- Gingival overgrowth into the preparation.

- An overbuilt proximal contour. This can be detected with dental floss. Stabilize the restoration with a finger and attempt to floss the contact. A shiny facet on the contact may indicate where metal should be removed with a green stone or small sandpaper disc. Where it is difficult to detect exactly where to disc, paint the contact area with a thin layer of graphite and water or use a proprietary spray developed for this purpose; dry the contact and insert the restoration. On removing the restoration the precise contact point will show as an area of metal where the graphite or spray has rubbed off. Metal should be removed from the contact until floss will just pass.

- If the restoration will not seat, distortion of the wax pattern or the impression is the likely cause. The fit surface of the casting should be carefully re-examined under magnification to see if there are any shiny areas which might give an indication of the site of an undetected blob on the casting. The preparation should then be re-examined for undercuts that could have caused the distortion. It is obviously preferable to avoid this situation as it is time-wasting and expensive.

If the marginal fit is good but the contact point is inadequate, this can be re-established by adding metal solder at the appropriate region.

Once the casting is seated the sponge should be removed and the occlusion checked in all excursions of the mandible. Articulating paper should be used to show initial contacts. Before removing the inlay to adjust these, the butterfly sponge should be replaced. When the occlusion has been adjusted the inlay should be removed, smoothed, and polished.

Finally, before cementation, the margins of the restoration should be burnished to the enamel. This can be done with hand instruments or rotating burnishers. The instrument should always be worked from the gold to the tooth.

Cementing the restoration

The inlay can be cemented with glass ionomer or zinc phosphate cement. In either case the quadrant must be carefully isolated and dried, and the cement mixed according to the manufacturer's instructions.

Zinc phosphate cement is mixed slowly to a creamy consistency. Glass ionomer cement is mixed rapidly to a slightly more viscous consistency. The cavity is filled with cement, using a flat plastic instrument, and the casting seated rapidly and firmly. The patient is asked to close firmly on a cotton-wool roll to apply a steady pressure while the cement sets. Excess cement should only be removed when the mix is completely set, taking particular care not to leave any flash of cement at the gingival margin (Fig. 10.7(e)).

Porcelain inlay

Modern porcelain inlays or onlays have an etched or at least a roughened fit surface. They are cemented with a composite luting cement to etched enamel or to a glass ionomer base. Thus, the retentive design of the cavity is less important than it is for a conventional cast metal inlay. There is still the need to remove caries and previous restorations, but in many cases a thick base of glass ionomer is placed, sometimes over a calcium hydroxide lining, and this serves the purpose of bonding together and strengthening the dentine remaining in the cusps. The porcelain inlay or onlay is primarily there to provide an occlusal layer which is resistant to abrasion and attrition.

The principles of the cavity design are that sufficient enamel or glass ionomer surface should be present for etching and that the margins should *not* be bevelled.

Figures 10.8 and 10.9 show typical preparations and restorations. The impression technique is the same as for indirect cast metal inlays and the alternative laboratory techniques, which are beyond the scope of this book, are briefly outlined on p. 162.

Special luting composite resins are used for cementation. The inlay is returned from the laboratory with the surface etched with hydrofluoric acid or simply left rough as a result of removing the refractory die by sandblasting. The tooth is isolated with rubber dam, the temporary inlay is removed, and the enamel and any glass ionomer cement which forms part of the preparation are etched, washed, and dried. The resin is then applied according to the manufacturer's instructions. With some luting cements the setting reaction is triggered by the application of a curing light, and the setting reaction then continues chemically. It is easier to remove excess cement before it finally sets. Once the cement is hard the rubber dam is removed and the occlusion checked with articulating paper and adjusted with fine diamond burs. Adjusted surfaces can be polished with composite finishing discs or with rubber wheels and points specifically designed for polishing porcelain.

Porcelain veneer

In most cases some tooth preparation will be necessary in order to accommodate the thickness of a porcelain veneer without making the tooth too bulky. Occasionally, the patient has had previous acrylic or composite veneers which have been added to the surface of the tooth and is therefore already accustomed to the appearance or greater bulk. In these cases little or no preparation of the enamel may be necessary once the existing veneers are removed. If preparation is required, a chamfer is produced at the gingival margin without penetrating the enamel. As the enamel tapers down to nothing at the cement-enamel junction only a fraction can be removed without risking the exposure of dentine. Enamel is also removed from the remainder of the buccal surface and into the contact area without going right through to the lingual side. The approximal finishing line is important. If it is left too far labially, it will show; if it is taken too far lingually, it will increase the difficulty of cleaning the junction and there is an increased risk of caries developing. The incisal edge may be left unprepared, or the incisal-buccal edge may be rounded off so that the veneer extends over it.

Impression techniques are again similar to the indirect cast metal inlay, although occlusal records are less important because these restorations should not be made where there is substantial occlusal contact on the restoration. An additional stage is the selection of the correct colour of porcelain using an appropriate shade guide. Temporary restorations are not usually needed. Again, the laboratory stages are outside the scope of this book. Porcelain veneers can be made by the fused porcelain powder techniques or by the casting technique (see p. 162).

In cementing the finished veneer it is important to achieve the correct colour. As well as choosing the correct porcelain shade, this is done by trying in the veneer using a non-setting trial cement which is available in a variety of shades. With thin porcelain veneers the colour of the cement has a considerable influence over the appearance of the final restoration.

Once the correct shade of cement has been chosen, the tooth and facing are washed and dried and the tooth is isolated and etched. The same shade of setting cement, usually a lightly filled resin-based cement, is then applied to the facing and

(a)

(b)

(c)

(d)

Fig. 10.8 (a) An MOD amalgam restoration in the lower second premolar tooth. Part of the lingual cusp has fractured off.
(b) The tooth prepared for an MOD porcelain inlay. A glass ionomer lining has been placed.
(c) The completed porcelain inlay on the die. This inlay was made in the laboratory on a refractory die and fired in the furnace.
(d) The porcelain inlay cemented in place. Note that the buccal margin of the restoration would be visible from the front of the mouth. This would have a better appearance in porcelain than in amalgam.

(a)

(b)

(c)

(d)

(e)

(f)

Fig. 10.9 (a) The unsatisfactory appearance of the first premolar tooth is due to the failed amalgam and the discoloration of the buccal cusp by the amalgam.
(b) The tooth has been prepared for an MOD porcelain inlay. The second premolar has also been prepared for a crown.
(c) A glass ionomer lining has been placed.
(d) The completed porcelain inlay improves the appearance of the buccal surface.
(e) The occlusal view. This inlay was made at the chairside by the Cerec machine.
(f) The Cerec machine. A small video camera on the left records a picture of the prepared tooth at the chairside. The shape of the inlay is designed with the aid of a computer built into the machine and then the porcelain inlay is milled from a block of porcelain in a small milling machine to the right.

(a)   (b)

(c)   (d)

Fig. 10.10 (a) An instanding discoloured upper lateral incisor tooth. The tooth is not vital and has been apicected, as has the central incisor. The central incisor already has a crown.
(b) A cast porcelain veneer. Note the translucency.
(c) The etched enamel surface. Note that this tooth did not need any preparation as one of the purposes was to build out the contour of the tooth.
(d) The completed porcelain veneer.

(a)   (b)   (c)

Fig. 10.11 (a) Tetracycline-stained teeth which had been treated with acrylic veneers several years ago. The margins of the veneers had begun to break down, making it difficult for the patient to clean and producing the gingival inflammation which can be seen. These teeth have now been prepared for porcelain veneers.
(b) Hi-Ceram porcelain veneers made on refractory dies. Note that they are opaque to disguise the underlying colour of the teeth.
(c) The completed porcelain veneers.

the facing is seated. The excess cement is removed and the cement is allowed to set. Most cements are initiated by a curing light.

Once any final adjustments have been made and the margins have been checked, the patient must be shown how to brush and floss to maintain the margins of the facing as plaque-free as possible, thus avoiding approximal caries and gingival inflammation (Figs. 10.10 and 10.11).

FURTHER READING

McConnell, R. J. Boksman, L., and Gratton, D. R., (1986). Etched porcelain veneers. *Rest. Dent.* **2,** 124–31

McLean, J. W., (1988). Ceramics in clinical dentistry. *Br. Dent. J.* **164,** 187–94

Smith, B. G. N. Wright, P. S., and Brown, D. (1994). *The clinical handling of dental materials* (2nd edn). Butterworth Heinemann, Oxford.

PART III

MONITORING AND MAINTENANCE

11 The long-term management of patients with restored dentitions

INTRODUCTION

Dental care involves more than the treatment of the consequences of disease. It concerns preventing disease, repair when necessary, and monitoring the restored state to ensure that health is maintained. Artifical restorations need to be checked regularly and occasionally repaired or replaced.

The dentist who has not seen his or her work fail over the years is myopic, peripatetic, or very young. It is appropriate to be critical about one's own operative work, continually seeking ways to improve. However, it is important not to be unfairly critical of the work of others, if only because we do not know the circumstances in which the restoration was done. Such criticism often betrays inexperience or arrogance. It is salutary to replace a restoration that has been condemned as faulty, only to produce a new restoration with just as many, if not more, faults. Preclinical operative dentistry is difficult, but when the manikin turns into a real person with fears, aspirations, and a small wet wriggling mouth, the difficulties are compounded.

Fig. 11.1   The enamel around the amalgam in the upper first molar is discoloured. This discoloration could be due to caries or corrosion of the amalgam. Since the discoloured area is so extensive, it is likely to indicate caries, which may be residual (the dentist left it in the first place) or recurrent (new caries).

THE WAYS IN WHICH RESTORATIONS FAIL

Restorations commonly fail in one of two ways: new disease or technical failure. This failure may be minor, requiring only monitoring or repair, or it may necessitate replacement of the restoration.

New disease

Caries and tooth wear

Placing a restoration in a tooth does not confer immunity on the tooth, and new disease may occur either around a restoration or on another aspect of the tooth (Figs. 11.1–11.4). This principle is particularly important with respect to caries and tooth wear. For this reason it is just as important to diagnose the cause of the disease and attempt to institute preventive measures as it is to restore the tooth tissue.

Pulpal problems

Heavily restored teeth are liable to pulpal inflammation. The pulp of a carious tooth which was vital at the time of restoration may still undergo necrosis as a result of either the original disease or damage from the operative procedures to restore it.

Fig. 11.2   A cavitated carious lesion is present at the cervical margin of the restoration in this molar.

Fig. 11.3 Caries is present beneath the restoration in the lower first molar. There is a large ledge of amalgam present on the mesial aspect of the upper first molar. This is a plaque trap and is probably responsible for the periodontal disease and mesial bone loss as well as the caries.

Fig. 11.4 There has been further tooth wear around the amalgam and gold restorations which are now 'proud' of the original tooth surface.

Fig. 11.3

Fig. 11.4

Fig. 11.5 A periapical radiograph of a heavily restored lower second premolar. A periapical area is present and the tooth does not respond to an electric pulp test.

Fig. 11.6 A soft vinyl mouth-guard.

Fig. 11.7 A periapical radiograph of a well-restored upper first molar which was excessively mobile due to bone loss caused by periodontal disease.

Toxins from the necrotic pulp result in inflammation of the periapical tissues and radiographic change (Fig. 11.5). Thus teeth with necrotic pulps should be root filled to prevent infection.

Trauma

Similarly, restoration of traumatized teeth will not prevent further trauma, although the use of a soft vinyl mouth-guard (gum shield) in those playing contact sports helps to prevent further injury. These can be made on study models, using a vacuum moulding machine and a sheet of soft plastic (Fig. 11.6).

Periodontal disease

Operative dentistry may also 'fail' for periodontal reasons. The tooth in Fig. 11.7 had been well restored recently, but periodontal disease and bone loss have now progressed to the stage where the tooth has to be extracted for the patient's comfort. This emphasizes that each examination of the dentition must include a thorough periodontal examination.

Technical failure

There are several technical reasons why restorations may be judged to have failed.

Fractured restorations

Fractured restorations are important, particularly those where the fractured pieces remain in place (Fig. 11.8) since this invites recurrent caries. Frequently, however, part of the fractured restoration is lost. The tooth may be symptomless or the patient may notice sensitivity to hot and cold, food packing, or a sharp edge with the tongue. Wherever a fractured restoration is to be replaced it is important to determine why the restoration has fractured. There is often a fault in the cavity preparation, such as too thin a restoration in a high-stress-bearing area, or the occlusion may have been incorrectly adjusted, and such errors must be corrected if the new restoration is to last.

Marginal breakdown

A particular problem with amalgam restorations is the phenomenon of marginal breakdown or fracture which is often referred to as *ditching* (Fig. 11.9). As early as 1895, G. V. Black noted this appearance and attributed it to deformation of the filling material under the stress of mastication. Recent research has confirmed this observation and has shown that the amalgam alloys with the lowest creep rate have the lowest incidence of marginal breakdown. Modern alloys with a higher copper content show a significant reduction in creep in comparison with previous alloys and are more resistant to corrosion. Since it has also been suggested that the

Fig. 11.8   **Fig. 11.9**

Fig. 11.8 A large amalgam restoration is present in the upper first molar. A distal part of the restoration fractured and was lost. A temporary zinc oxide and eugenol dressing is in place. The amalgam is also fractured mesially, with the fractured piece remaining in place. This invites recurrent caries in this tooth. A distal carious lesion can be seen in the premolar, shining up through the marginal ridge.

Fig. 11.9 Ditched amalgam restorations.

mechanism of marginal fracture is related to corrosion, alloys with a high copper content are likely to show improved marginal adaptation, and clinical trials have confirmed this. However, ditching may be reduced by attention to detail in cavity preparation. The amalgam-margin angle must exceed 70 degrees (see pp. 52 and 114) since angles less than this are prone to fracture.

While ditching is the main cause of marginal breakdown with amalgam restorations, cast restorations which are short of the margin were almost certainly 'short' when originally fitted since cast gold or or other metal does not deteriorate in this way. Immediately after cementation the gap between the casting and tooth would have been filled with cement. However, cements dissolve slowly in the oral fluids, and this may result in a space developing between the restoration and the tooth over a period.

Tooth fracture

Unfortunately, tooth fracture, especially loss of a cusp, is common (Fig. 11.10). Fractured cusps have often been weakened by the cavities for large amalgam restorations but this is not invariably the case. It is difficult to know which weakened cusps are liable to fracture and should be protected with cuspal coverage cast restorations or by adhesive intracoronal restorations, although examination of the occlusion will help.

It is not only caries that is to blame for cusp fracture. Since the advent of the airotor it is only too easy to overcut cavities. It is sometimes necessary to replace restorations a number of times over the years, and research has shown that occlusal cavities are often enlarged by an average of 0.6 mm in width each time that a restoration is replaced and thus, after a number of replacements, there is simply no tooth left.

Fig. 11.10 Part of the mesio-buccal cusp of the lower second molar has fractured adjacent to an amalgam restoration.

Diagnosis of cracked cusps

The diagnosis of cusp fracture is easy when the cusp has fallen off (Fig. 11.10). Before this actually happens, however, the patient may experience pain but often finds it remarkably difficult to locate this to a particular tooth. The patient will frequently complain of sensitivity to hot and cold and discomfort on biting. Even on clinical examination it is often difficult to pinpoint which tooth is causing the pain, but a fibre-optic light or disclosing solution may assist the diagnosis by making the crack easier to see. Lateral pressure on the suspect cusp may also help by producing a sensitivity that mirrors the patient's symptoms.

Defective contours

A *defective contact point* is often an immediate cause of failure of a new restoration (Fig. 11.11), and the patient may return to the surgery complaining of food packing.

In contrast, *overhanging margins*, which are particularly likely to occur gingivally, are only noticed by fastidious flossers. This failure is often not noticed by patient and

Fig. 11.11 A defective contact allowing food packing. The likely cause in this instance is mesial movement of the upper first molar following extraction of the upper second premolar.

dentist until new bite-wing radiographs are taken, and then the overhang is only too obvious (Fig. 11.12). Since overhanging margins are difficult to clean, they encourage plaque stagnation and therefore periodontal disease and caries.

Occlusal wear is well resisted by gold and amalgam but was a frequent cause of failure in the first generation of posterior composites (Fig. 11.13). The newer materials described in this book are claimed to be better in this respect and the results of clinical trials are promising.

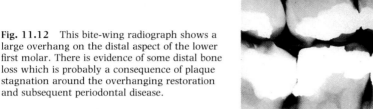

Fig. 11.12 This bite-wing radiograph shows a large overhang on the distal aspect of the lower first molar. There is evidence of some distal bone loss which is probably a consequence of plaque stagnation around the overhanging restoration and subsequent periodontal disease.

Fig. 11.13 Occlusal wear and marginal staining of the posterior composite in the lower first molar.

Fig. 11.12   **Fig. 11.13**

Appearance

Where the appearance of a restoration is important, deterioration in the colour match of the restoration with the tooth is an important cause of failure, often noticed by the patient as well as the dentist (Fig. 11.14). This problem is most common with the tooth-coloured restorative materials but can occur with amalgam restorations, where corrosion products may progressively discolour the rest of the tooth (Fig. 11.15). Unfortunately, it can be difficult for the clinican to differentiate staining due to corrosion from staining due to recurrent caries (Fig. 11.1). Recent research has shown colour change in the enamel adjacent to an amalgam restoration to be a poor predictor of recurrent caries, and the authors would rarely replace such a restoration, particularly if the margin was well adapted.

Fig. 11.14 A discoloured anterior composite on the mesial aspect of the upper left lateral incisor. The patient requested that this restoration should be replaced to improve its appearance.

Fig. 11.15 Corrosion products around the amalgam on the distal aspect of the upper right canine. The crown is discoloured and the patient is concerned by the appearance.

Fig. 11.14   **Fig. 11.15**

Failure of retention

A complete failure of retention is where the restoration is either lost or loose in the cavity. The latter invites recurrent caries (Fig. 11.16).

ACCEPTABLE AND UNACCEPTABLE DETERIORATION OR FAILURE

Research has shown that wide variation occurs between dentists in deciding which restorations have failed and should be replaced. In addition, the reasons for failure given by clinicians are subjective and very variable. These are uncomfortable findings which have disturbed the profession, but they are not altogether surprising. Dental students will probably not be surprised because they become used to variation in diagnosis and treatment planning among their teachers. The perspicacious dental student will realize that a treatment plan may have more to do with the attitude of the teacher with respect to when to restore caries or replace a restoration than the amount of disease with which the patient presents. This variation is inevitable when many factors, some of them poorly understood, are involved, and where additional research findings and clinical experience influence dentists at different rates.

Bias will also be contained within these pages. Many textbooks of operative dentistry do not address these questions which, in view of the confusion which exists within the profession, is understandable. The subject is obviously fraught with danger and the rest of this section must be regarded with healthy scepticism.

The patient's perception of the problem

The patient's opinion can and should influence the dentist's advice. The patient shown in Fig. 11.14 was unhappy with the appearance of the composite restoration; therefore this restoration, which was otherwise acceptable, was replaced. Some patients would be prepared to accept this appearance.

Similarly, the fractured cusp shown in Fig. 11.10 caused discomfort, as did the food packing occasioned by the defective contact seen in Fig. 11.11. In each case these restorations were replaced. The patient requested a tooth-coloured crown to deal with the staining around the amalgam in Fig. 11.15. Since considerable further destruction of the tooth would have been needed, this was not considered to be in the patient's best interest, and it was agreed that the amalgam should be replaced by a posterior composite.

Sometimes dentist and patient do not reach agreement because the dentist cannot accept that the patient's request is in his or her best interest. When this happens, they should agree to differ and part company. On no account should a dentist be persuaded to carry out treatment which he or she believes to be ill-advised. Not only is this unethical, but it is cases like this that subsequently may go wrong and can result in litigation.

The dentist's assessment of the effect of technical failure

The patient is often unaware of technical failure. The fractured restoration in Fig. 11.8 and the loose restoration in Fig. 11.16 were causing no symptoms but both were replaced because of the danger of development of secondary caries. However, Fig. 11.17 shows an occlusal amalgam with one small part fractured away. The cavity is very shallow (probably the cause of the fracture), easy to clean, and symptomless. Such a restoration might be left since its replacement with amalgam would result in the destruction of further sound tooth substance. However, a sealant restoration could be considered.

The ditched restorations shown in Fig. 11.9 also should not be replaced automatically. Ditched restorations should be accepted and put under review. This approach is particularly applicable in mouths which are not caries-prone. Replacement restorations frequently contain the same in-built errors as their predecessors. However, where a margin is severely ditched, so that it will admit the tip of a periodontal probe, plaque accumulation and therefore caries is encouraged. In this case it may be logical to repair only that part of the restoration, concentrating on improving it. If amalgam is used for the repair, a small retentive cavity is

Fig. 11.16 The amalgam restoration in the lower premolar has fractured. The pieces are in place, the tooth is symptomless and the patient is unaware that anything is wrong. The restoration should be replaced since this invites recurrent caries.

Fig. 11.17 An occlusal restoration is present in the lower first molar. The mesial portion of the amalgam has fractured, probably because the cavity is very shallow. Since the area is caries-free, easy to clean, and symptomless, this restoration does not have to be replaced yet. It would probably have been better to restore this tooth initially with a sealant restoration. If the amalgam does eventually have to be replaced, it would be advisable to consider replacing it with a sealant restoration. The fissures on the lingual side of the occlusal surface (top of the picture) are already stained, suggesting early caries at the base of the fissures.

prepared. Alternatively, cermet can be used, in which case a ditched crevice is prepared as for a glass ionomer fissure sealant.

Unfortunately, it is common to see ledges on amalgam restorations on bite-wing radiographs. These ledges usually cause plaque accumulation and gingival inflammation. Bleeding on gentle probing with a pocket measuring probe is evidence of this inflammation. Usually the ledge should be removed (see p. 188) or the restoration replaced to aid plaque control.

Secondary or recurrent caries

The diagnosis of secondary caries can be difficult. In one laboratory study dentists decided whether there was caries around restorations in extracted teeth before they were sectioned. The teeth judged as showing secondary caries in the simulated clinical examination did not always correspond to those which were found to be carious when sectioned. Some of the difficulties in the diagnosis of secondary caries become easier to understand if the histology of the early lesion is considered (see p. 8).

Caries can occur in the surface enamel next to the restoration. A cavity in this position can usually be seen unless it is on the approximal surface. However, leakage between the restoration and the tooth can result in caries of the cavity wall with spread beneath the restoration. Until the surface of the tooth either discolours or cavitates, this process may be difficult to detect.

In addition, the implication of the diagnosis must be considered. The problem is not so much whether *there is caries*, but whether *there is active caries* and whether this should be managed by preventive measures or operative intervention.

There are several visible signs of recurrent caries around a restoration. A white or brown spot on the tooth surface should be noted and managed preventively rather than operatively. However, a cavitated carious lesion adjacent to a restoration (Fig. 11.2) should usually be managed operatively as well as preventively, since the cavity is an obvious plaque trap and it is unlikely that the disease can be arrested.

Discoloration around restorations with clinically satisfactory margins is particularly difficult to interpret. With amalgam, this colour may be caused by corrosion products, and distinguishing this from caries is difficult (Figs. 11.1 and 11.15). Alternatively, a large amalgam restoration may discolour dentine without caries being present (Fig. 11.18). Recent research indicates that colour change may be irrelevant to the diagnosis of active secondary caries but may imply an arrested lesion. It seems possible that this appearance represents residual caries, left when the cavity was originally prepared, that has subsequently taken up stain. Thus, it is suggested that staining should rarely trigger the decision to replace a filling.

Fig. 11.18 A new amalgam restoration. Note how the amalgam discolours the tooth. In a few years time it may be difficult for another dentist to judge whether this discoloration represents the amalgam, corrosion products, or recurrent caries. (Compare with Fig. 11.1.)

However, all these decisions will be influenced by the caries status of the patient, since recurrent caries is more likely in the caries-prone mouth. In addition, where a dentist is dubious about a number of restorations a decision may be made to replace one of them. If this appears to show active caries beneath it, the dentist is more likely to decide to replace the others.

Caries beneath or adjacent to restorations is often visible on bite-wing radiographs. However, unless serial radiographs are available it may not always be possible to distinguish between new decay (recurrent or secondary caries) and decay left when restorations were placed (residual caries). Figure 11.19 shows caries beneath restorations which should be replaced.

Caries seen on radiographs at the cervical margin of the restoration (Fig. 1.20, p. 12) may be *root caries*, and this can be remarkably difficult to manage operatively (see p. 131). It may be preferable to try to arrest shallow lesions by preventive means. Frequent recall and careful examination is essential so that operative intervention can be carried out if the lesion progresses.

Fig. 11.19 A bite-wing radiograph showing recurrent caries distally in the lower second premolar and the lower first molar (arrows). There is occlusal caries beneath the restorations in the lower first and second molars (arrows).

MONITORING TECHNIQUES: RECALL AND REASSESSMENT

Monitoring dental health or restored health is one of the most important aspects of dental care. A course of treatment involving operative dentistry does not end once restorations have been completed. The aim of the initial course of treatment is to determine the level of dental disease, to find the cause, to arrest it by preventive means, and to provide restorations as required. However, these restorations do not themselves prevent further disease, but by restoring the integrity of the tooth surface they aid plaque control. This is why high-quality restorative dentistry is worth the effort, and shoddy work can be detrimental by encouraging plaque accumulation. However, it is the patient's efforts to control diet, to improve plaque control, and to apply other preventive measures which are of prime importance. It is patients who primarily control caries, not dentists.

Why then is it necessary to see patients again when all that appears to be required is compliance with simple preventive measures? To answer this, an analogy with the well-known relationship between smoking and lung cancer helps. Since this knowledge does not stop everyone smoking, why should the relationship between the frequency of sugar intake and caries modify patient's diet? Patients vary both in their susceptibility to the disease and in the lengths to which they are prepared to go to prevent it. However, preventive advice may be more readily accepted if it is regularly reinforced. Thus dentists recall their patients to repeat and modify any relevant preventive advice, to detect any new disease sufficiently early for preventive measures to arrest it, and to detect and repair technical failure. In addition, early disease is monitored to see whether preventive measures are being effective. This applies equally to caries, tooth wear, and periodontal disease.

Frequency of recall

How frequently should patients be seen for reassessment? This depends partly on the natural history of the disease. For example, teeth are most susceptible to enamel caries when they first erupt, and in older individuals exposed root surfaces are more susceptible than enamel. It also depends on the susceptibility of the individual to the various dental diseases and the success or otherwise of their preventive efforts; there is no general rule that can be applied to all. However, it is useful to have some guide, commonly accepted by patients, to ensure that individuals with a high risk of disease do not delay a recall visit for so long that there is a danger of irreparable damage.

For many years it has been accepted that patients should come to the dentist every six months. No strong scientific case can be found in favour of this period but equally there is no scientific case for altering it. It is the result of clinical experience and may be seen as a 'good average'. However, dentists should modify the recall interval according to the individual patient's disease pattern. Thus, a patient who initially presents with rampant caries or extensive periodontal disease might be advised to return at three-monthly intervals following the completion of treatment. However, a six-, nine- or twelve-month recall interval might be appropriate for individuals initially presenting with less rapidly progressing conditions. Regular, usually six-monthly, recall is particularly important where early carious lesions and mechanically imperfect restorations have been treated preventively or observed. Only with frequent monitoring is it ethical for a dentist to adopt this non-invasive approach when in doubt. The six-month or annual recall interval is also appropriate for the monitoring of tooth wear which appears excessive for the patient's age.

The recall assessment

The recall visit follows a pattern similar to the initial assessment described in Chapter 2. The history will concentrate on what has happened since dentist and patient last met. For instance, it is important to recheck the medical history carefully, but questions about past dental history need not be asked again except to check that no other dental treatment has been provided in the interim. When the clinical examination is carried out particular attention is paid to areas noted as important or specifically requiring monitoring. Thus, where suspect restorations or early carious lesions have been put on probation, a careful check of these is required (Figs. 11.20 (a) and 11.20 (b)).

Fig. 11.20 (a) A bite-wing radiograph showing an early distal carious lesion on the upper second premolar. Preventive advice was given and the rough amalgam on the mesial aspect of the upper first molar was smoothed with a linen strip to aid plaque control and flossing by the patient. A new radiograph was taken after six months to check that the lesion had not progressed.
(b) A bite-wing radiograph of the same area taken 18 months later. The carious lesion has apparently arrested.

(a)   **(b)**

The vitality of heavily restored teeth should be checked, paying particular attention to those where direct or indirect pulp caps were placed at the last visit.

Study casts are of particular assistance in monitoring the rate of tooth wear (Fig. 11.21). It is easier to compare two sets of casts than original casts with the current clinical picture.

The recall visit is in many ways one of the particular pleasures of the profession. When dentist and patient first meet they know very little about each other, but as the years pass they became better acquainted. Both dentist and patient often come to expect what will happen at the recall visit; perhaps a check that all is well and catching up on a year's news of family and work events. However, there is a trap here for the unwary professional. It is all too easy to assume that the mouth is stable or to perform a perfunctory examination, perhaps missing signs of early root caries, bleeding on probing in some areas, a sinus discharging over a non-vital tooth, or even an early malignancy. Attention to detail is vital.

If, as a result of proper history, examination, and special tests, treatment is required, the dentist should differentiate between that caused by essentially preventable disease and that occasioned by mechanical, aesthetic, or functional defects. The former require the patient's active co-operation in further preventive action.

Fig. 11.21 Two study casts showing progressive tooth wear. There was a three-year interval between the two impressions.

TECHNIQUES FOR REMOVAL, ADJUSTMENT, AND REPAIR

Up to now the operative part of this text has considered cavity designs unfettered by the presence of old restorations. Some mouths are already restored, and dentists currently spend more time replacing existing unsatisfactory restorations than treating new carious lesions.

Amalgam

Amalgam is a relatively easy restorative material to remove. An appropriate size and shape of Beaver but (see p. 98) is used in the airotor, and is inserted into the middle of the restoration and moved towards the cavity walls. The restoration can generally be removed with this bur but small fragments of amalgam may be left attached to the cavity walls and over the pulp; these are then broken away from the wall or floor with an excavator. Removing amalgam in this way avoids unnecessary overcutting of the cavity. No attempt should be made to 'freshen up' the margins, and the cavity should only be extended where caries dictates, where it has proved to be unretentive, or where the margin requires modification for other reasons such as chipped enamel or incorrect cavo-surface angle. Old lining material need not be removed unless caries has spread underneath it or the patient has symptoms of pulpitis and the operator wishes to look for an exposure.

It is often possible to repair an amalgam restoration, and this can be preferable to its complete removal where a single area requires extension or replacement. In these circumstances, removal and replacement of the entire restoration may introduce new faults.

Similarly, where new disease on another aspect of the tooth necessitates extension of a restoration, consideration should always be given to retaining part of the original filling. Exactly the same argument applies to restorations where part of the tooth fractures away. The original restoration may well be retained and a new cavity designed alongside and within it (Fig. 11.22). However, there is a need for some mechanical retention (such as a lock) between the new and the old filling. This technique can be particularly useful where pins are present in the original restoration. It is very difficult to remove such a restoration leaving the pins intact. If the pins are cut off when the restoration is removed, new pin sites will have to be found and this is difficult and risky for the pulp and periodontal ligament.

A decision to repair rather than replace a restoration should always be reviewed during the repair. If the initial cavity preparation reveals caries beneath the existing restoration, it should be removed completely.

The possibility of replacing small failed amalgam restorations with composite or glass ionomer – composite layered restorations should be considered. For example, they should be considered for the replacement of the restorations shown in Fig. 11.1, the first premolar in Fig. 11.9, and the canine in Fig. 11.15 (where it was in fact used). Composite could also be used for the premolar in Fig 11.16, particularly if the cause of the amalgam fracture was that the cavity was too shallow. In this instance a composite could be placed without deepening the cavity, whereas this would be necessary for a replacement amalgam.

Fig. 11.22 A large pinned amalgam restoration (two pins) was present in this upper first molar. The disto-buccal cusp fractured. The original amalgam is satisfactory and if it is removed two good pin sites will be lost. For this reason a third pin has been inserted and the amalgam will be repaired to serve as the base for a complete gold crown.

Composite and glass ionomer cement

Tooth-coloured filling materials are not as easy to remove as amalgam because the colour of the composite or glass ionomer cement is more difficult to distinguish from the tooth when under the water spray. Use of an airotor is again obligatory and small tungsten carbide or diamond burs may be chosen. The technique is identical to that with amalgam except for the following:

- The materials should not be chipped away from the enamel or dentine walls because these materials are adhesive and the forces may fracture the enamel at the cavity margins.

- The operator should stop frequently and the dental nurse should dry the tooth. A colour difference between tooth and and composite will now be easier to see.

Repair of these materials is an accepted technique as the new filling bonds to the old with adequate strength in some clinical situations. Where new material is to be added to old, it is important to cut some of the old material away to produce a clean surface for bonding. Where a restoration is subject to occlusal stress it is usually better to replace it.

Cast metal and ceramic restorations

These restorations can be time-consuming and tedious to remove. An appropriate size of Beaver bur in an airotor handpiece is the instrument of choice for cutting cast metal, and diamond burs should be used for ceramic restorations. It may be possible to divide the restoration and then use an excavator or flat plastic to break the cement seal, allowing the pieces to be removed individually. Great care should be taken not to fracture the tooth when removing an intracoronal restoration.

A small localized marginal discrepancy in an inlay caused either by an area of new decay or a lack of fit of the original restoration can be repaired by preparing a cavity adjacent to the inlay and restoring it with glass ionomer cement, composite, or amalgam.

Removal of ledges

It is very easy to produce a ledge of restorative material overhanging the gingival margin cervically. Careful matrixing, wedging, and early carving of this critical area will help to avoid this fault. Despite care, ledges may sometimes be created and discovered on a subsequent bite-wing radiograph (Fig. 11.12) Alternatively, the error may present as bleeding of the gingiva on probing as a result of plaque stagnation.

Buccal and lingual ledges are relatively easy to remove with fine tapered tungsten carbide or diamond finishing burs (see p. 100) but since these also cut the tooth easily, great care must be taken. Proximal ledges on tooth-coloured restorative materials can often be removed with abrasive strips, although where such ledges are large it may be less traumatic to the gingival margin and quicker to remove and replace the entire restoration or part of it.

Proximal ledges on amalgam restorations can be more difficult to remove. Sometimes the ledge is accessible to trimming with a flame-shaped steel finishing bur or metal abrasive strip. Alternatively, a special handpiece (Eva), designed specifically for the task, can be used (Fig. 11.23). This has a reciprocating (in-and-out) movement rather than revolving action. Small triangular wedge-shaped points, coated with abrasive on one side, are used in the handpiece to grind away the ledge. However, even when this is successful the remaining amalgam is often porous because it was not properly retained and condensed when it was being packed, and so, with extensive ledges, particular attention should be paid to wedging and trimming when the restoration is being replaced.

Fig. 11.23 An Eva handpiece being used to remove a ledge on the mesial aspect of the lower first molar.

SURVEYS OF RESTORATION FAILURE RATE

It is tempting for the student or dentist to regard his or her restorative work as permanent, but the work of others as less so. Before reaching for the airotor to remove existing restorations the dentist should pause to ask the following questions:

- How long has this restoration been in place?
- Why has it failed?
- How can future failure be prevented?

A number of surveys have been carried out on the longevity of restorations, many of these retrospectively by analysis of practice or dental school records. These show that 50 per cent of amalgam restorations last for eight to ten years. In studies of this nature the clinical decisions which condemned restorations or allowed them to survive were often made by the same dentist who placed them originally. This must influence the findings, as must the skill of the dentist whose records are examined.

Studies of this nature are often a testament to the ability of the individual practitioner, but are valuable in this respect because they show the best that might be hoped for.

A more representative picture of the situation nationwide would be gained by a longitudinal follow-up study of the dental care provided in the general dental service. Such a study is in progress in Scotland where the treatment of 720 adults is being followed. Results covering the first five years of this survey have been published, showing that 50 per cent of the routine amalgam and tooth-coloured restorations survived for less than five years.

This is a salutary finding, and one which should inspire student, teacher, and practitioner alike to work towards improved standards of diagnosis and prevention of dental disease, together with excellence in operative treatment.

FURTHER READING

Elderton R. J. (1983). Longitudinal study of dental treatment in the general dental service in Scotland. *Br. Dent. J.* **155**, 91–6.

Elderton, R. J. (1985). Six monthly examinations for dental caries. *Br. Dent. J.* **158**, 370–4.

Elderton, R. J. and Davies, J. A. (1984). Restorative dental treatment in the general dental service in Scotland. *Br. Dent. J.* **157**, 196–200.

Elderton, R. J. and Nuttall, N. M. (1983). Variation among dentists in planning treatment. *Br. Dent. J.* **154**, 201–6.

Kidd, E. A. M., Toffenetti, F., and Mjör, I. A. (1992). Secondary caries. *Int. Dent. J.* **42**, 127–38.

Merrett, M. C. W. and Elderton, R. J. (1984). An *in vitro* study of restorative dental treatment decisions and secondary caries. *Br. Dent. J.* **157**, 128–33.

INDEX